Contents

Acknowledgements

I would like to dedicate this book to every person who lives with persistent chronic pain. This book has reminded me we are strong, we are resilient and our story is one that needs to be told. To all my pain friends, far and wide, your support is a continuous blessing. I am so lucky to have a wonderful care bubble of health-care professionals who help me manage my chronic pain: my amazing GP Dr Penny Bleakley at Beechlawn Medical Centre, Monkstown, my pain specialist Dr Paul Murphy and his team Noelle and Kathryn, all the many nurses, doctors and experts on the pain management team in St Vincent's Hospital, the staff in Lloyds Pharmacy in Shankill, Dr Ashley Poynton, and last, but by no means least, Dr Graeme Sanders, who has given me endless advice and support.

I want to thank Vanessa Fox O'Loughlin for her enthusiasm, friendship and her belief in my story, which, along with Sarah Liddy's support and assistance, helped this book become a reality. Sincere thanks to all the wonderful team in Mercier Press for their guidance during the entire process. I would like to acknowledge Áine Toner, editor of *Woman's Way* magazine, who accepted my first article on chronic pain; without that first publication the seed for this book would never have blossomed. Thank you to Helen Goldin and Niamh Flynn for guiding me on my hypnosis journey. My healing relaxation that accompanies the book could not have manifested without the expertise of Paddy Gibbons and the kindness of Windmill Lane and Deborah Doherty in Number 4. To John Lindsay and the hardworking small team in Chronic Pain Ireland, thank you on behalf of all the members for the continuous work you do to highlight chronic pain.

I am blessed to have such wonderfully talented friends who have helped me throughout this journey: my dear friends Valerie Roe, Teresa Murray, Maureen Catterson, Ben Frow, Mark Cagney, Aisling Holly, Roisin Ni Mhorda, Suzie Carley and Olivia Leahy, thank you for having endless 'pain' chats. I was so lucky to work with some amazingly creative friends on the cover shoot: thanks to the wonderful Jenny McCarthy of Photosbyjen, to David Moran for his creativity, to Aimee Connolly for making me beautiful, and to Philip Rogers and the total hair care team who have managed my mane for over a decade! My brilliant stylist Ellen Redmond choose clothing from Avoca and Karen Millen – both have styled me for many years, such a treat. A special thank you to Avoca Kilmacanogue for allowing me to use its beautiful surroundings as a backdrop.

Heartfelt gratitude to all of my many close friends, too many to mention; I am so grateful for all the support while I dedicated myself to writing about chronic pain. It has taken longer than anticipated and has changed in direction along the way, because this is a story about my life in pain and sometimes the best-laid plans change because pain changes; thank you for your patience.

I am so appreciative of all my friends in St Anne's church in Shankill for the prayers and novenas, and of my alternative healers, Aidan Story and Carmel Howard. To my loving family Lavinia, Maria, Brian and of course my wonderful mum Marie, mother-in-law Mary and my second dad Pat, your endless love means the world to me.

One thing has been my rock – the love and support of my best friend and loving husband David and our beautiful daughter Brooke. You both remind me every day that pain will never win as my love for you both will always brighten my life, even on my darkest days.

Foreword

Dr Paul Murphy

The International Association for the Study of Pain (IASP) defines pain as 'an unpleasant sensory and emotional disorder due to actual or potential tissue damage or expressed in terms of such damage'. Throughout our lives, most of us are familiar with 'acute pain'. Whilst certainly unpleasant, this type of pain is often termed 'useful', as it serves a very important protective function. Chronic pain is typically defined as pain lasting in excess of twelve weeks. In many cases this can be considered 'useless' pain, as it serves no protective or beneficial purpose and instead leads to prolonged suffering. Chronic pain may arise from an initial injury or ongoing disease, but in some cases no identifiable cause can be found.

In recent years a paradigm shift has taken place, with a growing acknowledgement that persistent pain should be considered a disease entity in its own right. Prior to this, pain had primarily been considered to be a passive warning sign of an underlying disease process. Based on this model, the focus of healthcare professionals had been to identify this underlying cause and, by remedying it, relieve the painful symptom. We now accept that pain cannot always be regarded in this manner and that chronic pain is associated with a range of changes in nerve function, mood, cognition and social function.

Pain is therefore a profound personal and subjective experience. As there is no test that can objectively measure pain intensity and location, the pain sufferer and their healthcare professionals must work closely together to assess not only potential causes of pain, but also the impact of ongoing pain across a range of psychosocial domains.

In 2010, with 'The Declaration of Montreal', the IASP stated that access to pain relief should be considered a basic human right. Representatives and members from 129 countries turned their attention to the problem of unrelieved pain on a global setting. It was found that there was inadequate access to treatment for acute pain due to trauma and disease. It was also acknowledged that there remain major deficits in the knowledge of healthcare professionals regarding the mechanisms and management of pain.

Chronic pain, with or without diagnosis, is highly stigmatised and lacks appropriate recognition as a serious health problem in its own right that requires treatment akin to other chronic conditions. Many countries have no national policy at all or very inadequate policies regarding the management of pain as a health problem, including an inadequate level of research and education. Until recently 'Pain Medicine' has not been recognised as a distinct speciality with a defined scope of practice.

In 2010 the IASP declared that 'in recognizing the intrinsic dignity of all persons and that withholding of pain treatment is profoundly wrong, leading to unnecessary suffering which is harmful, we declare that the following human rights must be recognized throughout the world:

- Article 1. The right of all people to have access to pain management without discrimination.

- Article 2. The right of people in pain to acknowledgement of their pain and to be informed about how it can be assessed and managed.

- Article 3. The right of all people with pain to have access to appropriate assessment and treatment of the pain by adequately trained healthcare professionals.'

This book provides a wonderful insight into Andrea's journey through chronic pain and should act as a source of hope and encouragement for other pain sufferers.

Introduction

In December 2013 I took a phone call that would change my life for ever. Having spent more than half of my life looking for an explanation for the constant pain I have had since my teens, it suddenly seemed as if I might have an answer.

It was a Monday morning and I was sitting at my desk in TV3 feeling the pressure. I was in the middle of shooting a one-hour festive TV special called *Coming Home for Christmas*, and the show had to be filmed, edited and delivered on time to air on Christmas Eve. On top of this, I was guest presenting on *Midday*, a daytime girls-only chat show on TV3. I also had my radio work, a Saturday talk and music show on Sunshine 106.8, and some voice-over work. To add to this, I had volunteered to cover a few afternoon shifts on a charity station, Christmas FM. Finally, like everyone else, I had my festive shopping to do, Christmas parties to attend and all the preparation for Santa in our house. It was all go and I was wrapped up in it all.

I was checking the diary on my phone when a number flashed up. I recognised it instantly: St Vincent's Hospital. When I answered, to my surprise I heard my doctor's voice. Towards the end of the year I had been feeling unwell. I had suffered from 'back issues' for many years and the pain in my neck, shoulders and down my right arm was now constant and debilitating, so my doctor had scheduled an MRI scan to investigate further. I had been attending Dr Paul Murphy for many years and had never received a call from him, so perhaps I should have listened a bit more carefully when he started to speak and asked a few more questions, but I just said: 'Yes, yes, em … yes, OK, great, thank you, see you on Friday … bye.'

I did manage to scrawl down the words 'Chiari malformation, 1-2-3', and from what I remember, Dr Murphy said something about some degeneration showing up on the most recent MRI scan and then mentioned Chiari malformation 1. It was a rare condition, he said, and I had the mildest type, type 1, which meant that my brain was pressing downwards. Although it can be asymptomatic, he wanted to get it checked out. He then explained to me that he had called me personally because he didn't want me to be alarmed when he sent me the test results. He would also send them to my GP, and if I had any questions I could call him at any time. Moreover, I was booked in that week for a procedure with him, so we could discuss it then.

I hung up, almost not reacting. A colleague and friend was at my desk when I got the call and asked me if I wanted to talk about it over coffee. I said yes, and as I sipped my coffee he said, 'Now don't go googling it, that's the worst thing you can do!' I knew he was right, so I didn't at the time. I put it to the back of my mind.

I did, however, do something totally unplanned later that day. Without really thinking about it, I approached my line manager with a view to getting some time off in the new year. By the end of the week I had email confirmation that I could take three months' leave, starting in January. Knowing I would have this time off seemed to push me through that busy time. My pain level was very high, but knowing that some downtime was ahead was a real motivator.

So in January 2014 I took leave from TV3 to follow my own pain management programme. I knew my lifestyle needed some adjustment, but I wasn't quite prepared for the journey and massive changes that lay ahead. The process hasn't been easy and has involved lots of highs and some very dark lows, but one thing has anchored me along the way – the confidence to be an empowered patient. I have taken control of my own life, my own health. It has been a voyage of discovery, in which I have been guided by my desire and the belief that I can 'heal' myself back to perfect health, happiness and wellness. I followed my instincts on self-healing and as a result I have changed, my pain has changed, my whole life has changed. This book is the story of that journey.

My Story

1

Childhood

My earliest memory is of my mother and father's room. I am in a cot at the end of their bed and my brother is kicking the cot with his legs as he sits on the ground. This seems like a great game and I am laughing as I fall from side to side. Because I was the youngest in my family, I was doted on by my sisters and brother. Lavinia is the eldest and there is an eleven-year age difference between us. Then comes Maria, who is nine years older than me, and my brother Brian, who is four years older. Despite this, when I recall my childhood I always remember feeling a little bit different. I liked my own company. I played a lot on my own with my imaginary friends and spoke to Mother Mary, many angels and even saints! I had a vivid imagination and I enjoyed living in my own little world.

Part of the reason for my isolation was probably a hearing problem I had, which was only detected when I was about six or seven years old. As well as this, in some respects, from very early childhood I was always in a state of pain. I had more or less constant earaches or headaches, which meant I was in and out of Temple Street Children's Hospital. My first stay there was to have my tonsils removed. Next time it was to have my adenoids removed, and before long I was well acquainted with the hospital's ENT department. I had multiple operations on both ears, so hospital stays were fairly regular. The longest was probably around two weeks, and I remember feeling very lonely in there. It was only as I got older that I realised how difficult that time was for my mam. She had three older children at home – my sisters were in secondary school, my brother was still in junior school – and Dad was working, so she would often take the bus to the hospital to see me during the morning while the others were at school. I don't remember my sisters or brother ever visiting me.

My ward had a little nurses' station or medicine room in the corner, then a little corridor leading to the toilet with a large, white, free-standing bath. The ward had just five beds and looked onto a flats complex across the road. Every morning the nurses would set up little tables and chairs in the centre of the ward where we would eat our breakfast cereal. Sometimes we got hot milk, which I enjoyed a lot. I can still remember the distinct smell of hospital food, not always very pleasant, and I really enjoyed going home and having my mother's cooking – after a hospital visit she had a tradition of making me oxtail soup with fresh crusty bread.

I was in hospital so frequently I attended the little hospital school. I remember not knowing my ABCs and this seemed to be very troubling for the nun who was teaching us. I suppose because I wasn't hearing correctly, I wasn't learning. The school or playroom part of the hospital was at the top of a narrow stairwell – I have a vague recollection of falling down those stairs. I think I was quite clumsy, as on another occasion I fell out of my bed in the hospital.

With all my health problems I was always catching up when I returned to my own school. I know I had learning challenges with both reading and spelling, and I was put into a special class with a teacher called Miss Walshe. I was eight years old at this point. I loved her class as she made up little rhymes to help us remember our ABCs – this was the first time I remember reading. The first book we read was *Fantastic Mr Fox*. Once I understood how to read there was no stopping me. My favourite place as a child was the mobile library that came to our area once a week. I read so many wonderful books as a child and I will always be thankful to Miss Walshe, who fostered my love of reading and books. Luckily, she recommended that I should stay back and repeat a year in school so I could catch up academically, which I did.

Before Miss Walshe helped me with my reading and spelling, I don't remember being particularly bright as a child. In fact I remember getting into trouble for daydreaming or not listening, and I was often sent to sit at the nature table as punishment. I frequently sat there with a boy who ate crayons. However, I can clearly remember being able to lip-read quite easily as a child, and I feel I had a sixth sense, almost knowing things were going to happen before they did. One memory that stands out for me is telling some of my classmates that our beloved local priest, Fr Kearns, was going to die and go to heaven. I just said it very matter-of-factly; I think I may have even said it to the priest himself during a visit he made to our classroom. I didn't think too much about it, but very soon afterwards he did die and the whole school attended prayers for him in the church. One of my school pals told me that I had killed him because of what I had said, which frightened me and I was worried that I would get into trouble.

This wasn't the first time this had happened. A lovely old man, Mr O'Neill, who lived across the road from our house, died the day after I had a dream that he was being brought to heaven by a scary woman. Again I shared my dream and was aware that people thought the whole thing was spooky. I wonder if my poor hearing had anything to do with my extra sense, visions and dreams.

By the time I was twelve, both of my sisters were living in

the UK. This was before Skype and FaceTime, so I would write letters and give them to my parents to send to England. I really missed Lavinia and Maria; the house seemed a lot quieter and there was a sadness and a real sense of loss, for Mum especially. I remember often hearing her crying in those early days. It was a confusing and upsetting time for me as well, as I recall not feeling very involved in my eldest sister Lavinia's departure. I don't really remember anyone explaining the reasons for her leaving, as my parents didn't talk about it – I think they felt it might be too upsetting for everyone – and I didn't go to the airport so I never had a chance to say a proper goodbye. For the first time our family was fragmented and our unit, as I knew it, would never be the same again. This was during the 1980s, when many young people had to travel to find work, and, like so many others, my sisters never returned.

When my sister Maria decided to follow in her big sister's footsteps, I did go to the airport. She was 'emigrating' with my cousin so it was a big family affair and there was a grand send-off in Dublin Airport. This time it was much easier for me, as I was a little older and understood why she was leaving.

Not too many years later, my brother, Brian, would follow the same path. Both of my sisters still live in the UK, while Brian is in Hong Kong. Thankfully, technology makes it much easier to stay in touch these days.

Eventually I left primary school, my hearing troubles and, for a while, my pain behind. The operations seemed to have eased the pain and I left junior school having done very well academically. I was, on the whole, a very active, healthy teenager. I was involved in the parish Faith Friends programme, I played sport, was a member of the debating team, loved dancing and drama and even took up swimming. All during my childhood I was encouraged not to get water in my ears, as it would cause extra pain, but as a teenager I wanted to learn how to swim – and I did.

I can honestly say I really loved secondary school. I had the opportunity to really get involved in the school community and I have fond memories of my teachers and fellow students. In my final year at St Mary's Holy Faith in Killester I was even chosen as head girl, which was a great honour. For a large part of my secondary school life I was healthy, happy and full of life, and never missed a day – but, unfortunately, that would all change when I was fifteen.

2

Age Fifteen

After I turned fifteen in 1993, I woke up one morning feeling sick. I wasn't vomiting but I felt physically unlike anything I had ever felt before. I had no energy. As a rule, I very rarely went to the doctor, so, trying to gauge how serious it was, my mam said: 'Well, if you're really sick and too ill for school, you should go to the doctor with your dad.' Usually I would have said no, knowing that my dad would quiz me and I'd need to be really sick, but on this occasion I felt so unwell that I was happy to walk to the doctor's with him. By the time I got to the doctor's office I felt very weak. It was a bright, sunny day and the sunlight streaming through the window of the surgery made my head ache. Before I knew what was happening, I was getting into an ambulance. We stopped by the house to get some things for hospital and then I was lying on a gurney heading for Cherry Orchard Hospital. I had suspected meningitis.

I don't remember much of what followed. I became very sick, very quickly. I was put into an isolation room and spent much of the next four weeks on my own there. My dad visited me every day and brought my mam up every other evening. The hospital was two bus journeys from where we lived, so it was a long trek daily for my dad. He brought up a small radio so that we could listen to RTÉ 1 while he sat with me and as I lay listless in bed. At one point I hallucinated that Elvis was in the room. It must have been a very worrying time for my parents.

Finally, the decision was made to give me a spinal tap (a

lumbar puncture) to enable a definitive diagnosis of meningitis, a procedure that involves analysing the cerebrospinal fluid. My dad explained to me that a needle would be inserted into my back to take a sample of some fluid so the doctors could see what antibiotics they needed to give me. He told me to listen to the music and focus on the radio, to try to stay still and be brave.

The procedure, which was done in the middle of the night, seemed to take a long time and I remember lying at the edge of the bed just waiting for it to be over. I can still recall the first song on the radio – 'What's Going On' by 4 Non Blondes. However, the events of that evening aren't very clear, and my father, the only person who could truly confirm what actually happened, has since passed away. I do remember feeling terrible after they had finished, with lower back pain and a headache. Dad told me that this was normal. We never spoke about it afterwards; he said that I was very brave not to cry and the best thing was to forget about it and not to upset my mam by telling her about it.

As far as I know, I had viral meningitis linked to glandular fever, and I remained quite ill for some weeks. Lavinia and Maria both flew home to see me. Normally, it would have been really exciting for me to see my two sisters home again, but I couldn't even talk to them; I just remember them being in the room. Brian also came to visit, and he would sit in the room and draw. I would occasionally wake up and look for a sip of water, and he would try to cheer me up with pictures he had drawn while I was asleep.

After a few weeks of treatment, however, I felt like a different person. I had my energy back and was ready, even eager, to return to school. I think when I asked my dad to bring in my school-books, he knew I was almost ready to come home. The only worrying issue was that from then on I had persistent lower back pain and periodic headaches. At the time the doctors thought this was linked to my menstrual cycle, and I was told that after my illness I would feel tired and sore until I got stronger again.

As a teenager in a typical Irish family, I didn't talk to my parents about my periods. My sisters were away, so I couldn't confide in them, and after chats with friends I thought that everyone experienced lower back pain during their monthly cycle. So I didn't think I was any different and it seemed that the pain I felt was normal. In fact, when I went for a check-up with the same doctor who had ordered the ambulance for me to go to Cherry Orchard, and told him I had a very sore lower back, I was embarrassed to explain just how low it was – it was around my coccyx and I didn't want him to touch my bottom! He prescribed Ponstan painkillers for me to take when required.

When I had finished the Ponstan I asked my mam if I could go and get some more. Mam never had tablets in the house, so she totally disagreed with me taking them. She told me that everyone had growing pains and period pains and that it would get better, so I shouldn't keep taking tablets, I just needed to get on with it. As a result, I ended up buying Feminax myself and taking them almost daily for a number of years. I also didn't mention the pain again until I was involved in a snowboarding accident some years later.

9th December 1993

Dear Diary,

I have missed so much time from school I am feeling really under pressure about the Christmas exams. Mr Mulcahy told me not to get too stressed out about it and focus on catching up in time for the mocks. I am still exhausted all the time but I am so happy to be back in school. I have dropped out of basketball for the moment until I have my check-up with Dr Dwyne. I am looking forward to Christmas, I think Maria might be coming home which will be great. I am going to start getting the decorations down from the attic, maybe me and Brian will put up the tree this weekend. Roll on Christmas.

3

Age Twenty-Three

I met my husband, David, in Dublin when I was studying film and television in college. We met in Café en Seine in April 1998, a month before my twentieth birthday. It was the Easter bank holiday weekend and we spent the whole weekend together watching movies, eating ice cream and having lots of fun. I had some college work to hand in on the Tuesday and I was concerned about where I was going to type up my paper. I didn't have a computer or printer. To my amazement, David said I could type it up in his office on the bank holiday Monday. He worked in graphic design and he had gone to the same college as me, the Dublin Institute of Technology, so he knew the lecturers and offered lots of helpful advice. By the end of the weekend we were planning a trip to London. From the day we met we were inseparable and, before long, I had moved in with him. Life was really good.

After college I started work in Windmill Lane. I loved having my own money – and being able to spend it, too. In 2001, when I was twenty-three, David and I planned a long-haul trip. We both loved travelling and were enthusiastic snowboarders. This was to be our first snowboarding holiday alone together, as usually we went with a group. We were heading for Banff in Canada and we were both very excited about the trip.

On the day we arrived we spent most of our time renting out our equipment and organising our slope pass for the week. The soft, powdery snow was very different from what we had been used to in Europe. We took it easy in the afternoon and only did one or two smaller runs on the mountain, adjusting to the conditions and the slope.

On our second morning there we went up the mountain really early. We took a chair lift right up to the peak of the mountain, feeling very excited about our first full day on the slopes. For our first descent we decided to take different runs and meet at the bottom. The mountain was empty and we felt very pleased with ourselves at being the early birds and getting to carve the first fresh tracks into the snow.

I really enjoyed the freedom of boarding down the mountain, but as it was the first run, some parts were still a bit icy where it was shaded and the glare of the sun made it difficult to see properly. Without warning, while going at speed on my board, I caught an edge and fell forward, sliding quite a distance down the mountain. Immediately my wrist began to hurt and I lay there for a few minutes, hoping that someone would come to my aid. Eventually two skiers came down and picked up my glasses and hat, which had fallen off higher up the mountain. They didn't stop, just kindly put them beside me and were gone in a flash. I didn't have a mobile phone and I knew I had to get down and meet David, but it wasn't going to be easy. I managed to get up on the board and I went down the run on my heel edge, trying to avoid any flat areas. It took a while, and when I was almost at the end of the run I collapsed and waved wildly for David to come to my aid and take my boots off. I knew I hadn't the strength in my wrist.

I was pretty sure I had broken my arm or wrist and wanted to go to the hospital for an X-ray. However, David and the local mountain A&E team assured me that I would know if I had broken something, as the pain would be unbearable. I took some of my trusted Feminax, but reiterated that I thought I needed to get it checked out anyway. Although I was worried that I was wasting people's time, something told me I had seriously damaged my arm.

We arrived at the calm and lovely Mineral Springs Hospital in Banff. An X-ray confirmed a broken wrist and it was set in a cast. At this time I did mention an increased pain in my lower back. I felt pretty rough all over; it had been quite a spectacular fall and I seemed to bash myself a bit coming down the mountain, so extra pain was to be expected, but the pain in my back did seem a lot worse after the accident. I explained the situation to the very kind doctor in the hospital, who advised me to get a check-up and X-ray in Dublin, and said I should also mention the persistent lower back pain to my doctor.

I was given some anti-inflammatory tablets and was off the mountain for the rest of the trip. Despite the broken wrist and a lot of overall body pain from the fall, it was a great holiday. The anti-inflammatories made the pain bearable and I read book after book to pass the time during the day while David went snowboarding. We would meet for lunch every day and he would go back up on his own for a few more runs while I waited below.

Back in Dublin I went to Beaumont Hospital to have my wrist re-cast and get a new X-ray. Taking the advice of the doctor at Mineral Springs, I also went to see a GP, although at the time I didn't have a regular doctor. Our trusted family doctor, who had known me all my life, had retired, and I had only ever gone to a Well Woman Clinic in town for routine checks. I was generally very healthy and never had a reason to go to a doctor. So on this occasion I went to a medical centre in Dublin city centre. I explained about the accident and the lower back pain, but no explanation was forthcoming. I was prescribed Difene, which really helped with the pain and I went back to feeling pretty normal again. Although my lower back pain remained, it just seemed to be something I was going to have to live with.

Meanwhile, my mam was worried about all the tablets I was taking and was convinced that I had really hurt my back in the snowboarding fall. But, being young and busy, I ignored her advice to get a scan to have it checked out. I felt that I had recovered very well from the fall and I was doing fine. In the meantime, I arranged to visit my sister Maria and her family in the UK, so Mam spoke to Maria and urged her to echo her concerns, in the hope that if I wouldn't listen to her, I might listen to my sister.

During the visit I had unusually heavy and prolonged menstrual bleeding, coupled with lower back pain and some headaches, and, sure enough, my sister expressed her alarm at the number of tablets I was taking. I had asked her to buy some painkillers for me when she went to the shops, and a few days later I needed another packet. We had a heated discussion about my consumption of 'pills', and she was so concerned that she spoke to David and asked him to promise that he would make me seek out a medical expert in Dublin to discover what was going on.

The fact that Mam, Maria and David were all concerned made me sit up and take notice. I started to listen to them and decided that I needed to find out if it was 'women's problems' that had been causing this pain after all, or if there was something else going on. I also decided to look at alternative ways to improve my health.

August 2001

Andrea's things to do

Diet Diet Diet – Detox all week.

Pain-*free* Life

Dear Diary,

I haven't written for a while, I have been so busy after the holiday trying to settle back into work. After coming back from Maria's I have been really determined to try to sort myself out. I decided to get an allergy test done just in case my lower back pain is IBS, so tonight after work I went to Phibsboro for my second session of homeopathic acupuncture and to get the results of the tests.

The results are very interesting, it seems I am allergic to so many different things. So I need to write a food diary and basically eat only fresh, non-processed foods until next week's session. I feel very uneasy at the moment and I hate it when I feel like this. I still feel (well kinda) that there might be something more serious wrong with me. I am trying to stay positive and not get stressed about everything, but I feel like even writing down that I am worried is worrying. I need guidance, please let me be strong and find the answers I need. Maybe the pain is from constipation and eating all the wrong foods that my body can't process? Hoping when I write next some amazing new wonderful development will unfold that will give me energy and make me feel better. Feeling a little sore. Please God make me sleep. A x

4

Getting Help with 'Women's Problems'

When I got back to Dublin I tried to tackle my problems naturally and explored some homeopathic remedies, but things didn't really improve, so after much consideration I decided to seek advice from an expert. I made an appointment for Mount Carmel, a private hospital, to see a highly regarded gynaecologist. I felt really positive that I would finally get to the bottom (pardon the pun) of my lower back/coccyx pain.

I had a long consultation with a lovely doctor. We discussed at length my history and how I had been self-medicating with Feminax and had now started to use Solpadeine too. The doctor seemed very confident I had PCOS – polycystic ovary syndrome – and possibly endometriosis. She took some blood, did a number of physical tests and then an internal exam, and she seemed pretty confident that she had diagnosed me correctly. She also said that she was confident that she could reduce the pain. I was scheduled to have a scan of my ovaries.

Naturally I was happy to have a name for the pain. I felt really validated when she said, 'No matter what anybody tells you, the pain from endometriosis is real, we will take it seriously and help you, and you can help yourself, too, through diet.' So, while I was a little shocked that I might have these serious conditions, which can affect fertility, I felt I was in good hands.

Immediately, I went out to buy the books recommended by the doctor – *Endometriosis: A Key to Healing and Fertility through Nutrition* by Michael Vernon, and the *PCOS Diet Book* by Colette Harris, a nutritional approach for polycystic ovary syndrome. There was a lot to take in. I was very scared about what this diagnosis might mean for me as a woman. Would I be able to have a family? At this stage I had been going out with David for many years and we were in a strong, stable and loving relationship. I feared this would put a massive strain on us, so I wanted to do everything that I could to help myself and I really wanted to embrace whatever advice the books might give.

Being my usual proactive self, I started to see a Chinese herbalist, who treated me for PCOS and endometriosis. This involved many 'treatments' each week. I took some prescribed herbal tablets and daily drops, and started a strict diet – no sugar, no processed foods, no alcohol. I had to agree to completely stop my Feminax fix – all over-the-counter medication was banned. My body was a temple and I needed to detox. The herbalist felt that the toxins in my body might be causing my inflammation and pain. I was so desperate to get better, and so worried that I wouldn't be able to conceive, that I was prepared to do virtually anything. I was very vulnerable and during the next few months I spent a lot of money on drops, potions and various healers. Yet, while my new healthy approach to life did make me feel better, my pain was worse. In spite of my 100 per cent commitment to my diet and to detoxing, I wasn't coping very well; the pain was terrible and I wasn't able to manage it by diet alone.

I returned to Mount Carmel to see the doctor. When we spoke again about the signs and symptoms of endometriosis I was more convinced than ever that this was what I had. She asked me some questions about my symptoms and I appeared to have a lot – painful menstrual cramps, persistent pain in my pelvic area and lower back, pain with bowel movements, feeling fatigued. Then she mentioned difficulty getting pregnant. I had never been pregnant, but when she asked me what contraception I used, I had to be honest and say we didn't use contraception. This seemed to worry her. She quizzed me on the duration of our relationship. I think at that stage we had been together almost seven years and the fact we had never 'got caught' seemed to suggest that maybe we would have difficulty conceiving. All this combined gave the doctor the strong opinion that the next move for us should be to investigate and she recommended surgery.

So, before I could think about it, I was booked in for a laparoscopy, an operation in which a small cut is made below the belly button and a scope is inserted to take a look at the uterus, tubes and ovaries; as you can imagine, it isn't too pleasant. However, I told myself it would all be worth it. I would finally know what was the root cause of my lower back pain and the procedure would be one step closer to the pain-free life that I craved so much.

What happened next was a really low point for me. I simply wasn't prepared to hear from the doctor that she had found no evidence of endometriosis. Once again I was at a complete loss to know why I had this mysterious and persistent pain. I had trusted this doctor and I had had absolute faith in her when she told me my pain was caused by endometriosis. She had given me hope that we would sort this pain out. So when she said she couldn't find any evidence of the condition and offered no advice on what to do next I genuinely felt I was going mad. I had this terrible pain but was being told, 'You have nothing wrong with you.' Nobody, it seemed, could identify what was causing it.

I shared the news that the doctor had found nothing wrong with family and close friends, and I truly felt, at times, that my family was questioning exactly what was going on with me. I even doubted myself. Was I imagining the pain? I think that's when the word 'stress' came up a lot. At the time there were a lot of references in the media to 'yuppie flu' – a mysterious illness that seemed to affect younger working people and sapped them of their energy. I think my mam was convinced that's what I was suffering from. 'You're living your life in the fast lane!' she said. I couldn't deny it; I was always busy and my motto was 'work hard, play hard'.

I was more in need of answers than ever. I went to healers and massage therapists, I tried acupuncture and personal trainers who specialised in back problems. Everyone, it seemed, thought they knew what was wrong and had a solution. But nothing worked. I was still stuck with the pain, but had a lot less money in my pocket.

I was still working in Windmill Lane, where I had moved from visual post-production to sound, working alongside the legendary Paddy Gibbons, one of Ireland's most highly regarded sound engineers. I was the studio manager and busy all the time. I had also started doing one or two shifts a week hosting in one of Dublin's trendiest nightclubs – Lillie's Bordello. My shift started at eleven at night and I wouldn't get home until between 2 a.m. and 5 a.m. Remarkably, I always made it into Windmill Lane if I was working the next day.

The job at Lillie's came about in an odd way. I was a close friend of the club's hostess, Elaine Roddy. We were out to dinner one night when she got a call from another hostess who couldn't work. Elaine was really stuck and she managed to convince me to cover the shift. Before I knew it, I was part of the family, and we were a close-knit bunch, with Valerie Roe at the helm. The work was really easy, it was sociable, I was meeting people and having fun – with no expense and no hangover the next day!

I enjoyed being busy, I was young and I was working hard, but both jobs were really fun. It was during the roaring Celtic Tiger years, so the Windmill Lane expense account was being well used!

There was lots of client entertainment and I was very good at it; I was a bit of a party girl – but who isn't in their twenties? Our clients were creative types, and it was definitely not your nine to five office job. No one would think anything of getting a runner to go to The Dockers pub to order a couple of JDs and coke for a client who was in a long session. It also wasn't uncommon for people to be drinking and smoking (still legal in the workplace then) at the editing desk. It was all part of the creative process.

While I loved the fun side of working in the world of TV post-production, I did ask myself if it was perhaps too demanding. We started sessions in the studio before 8 a.m. and we wouldn't finish until 7 p.m. or later. Socialising was part of getting a gig, and there were frequent events and client dinners to go to; most evenings I was out and about. With all the work and partying, I began to think that maybe this mysterious pain could be related to my crazy, busy, demanding lifestyle. I was definitely burning the candle at both ends, so was Mam right?

In a way, I think I was almost testing my body to see just how much it could endure. Between working late nights and starting early mornings I was existing on four to six hours' sleep a night. Even when I wasn't working, sleep was always a problem because of the back pain, so in a way I felt I might as well be working, but I was running myself into the ground. So I had a ready-made excuse for the pain – it was easy to blame it on long hours at a desk, or standing for long periods wearing high heels, or dancing into the early hours! I was pushing myself and maybe, secretly, I wanted to keel over from exhaustion so a doctor would tell me to stop.

When I chatted about my back pain at work I found most people in the building had backache from long hours editing or mixing TV programmes. In a way it was easier to say to myself: 'Yes, my pain is directly linked to my work life.' Even taking my new painkiller of choice, Solpadeine, every day seemed to be the norm too. A client, who is now a close friend, started his day with a cocktail of three or even four of the effervescent tablets. I didn't feel I was any different.

Despite this, I did take a good look at my work environment and tried to see if I could make small changes that might benefit my mental and physical well-being. At the time I was largely desk-bound, always on the phone, booking sessions, doing accounts. Everything centred on the computer and the phone, and I usually ate lunch at my desk. I started to wonder if my pain was related to my office chair and my lifestyle. In the world of television post-production money is no object, and I needed the perfect chair to ensure that my back was supported. Windmill Lane were fantastic and very supportive about my request to work in an office with a positive back healthcare system for employees. One of my colleagues, Martin, researched and sourced the perfect ergonomic office chair, not just for me but for all the studio engineers as well. He thought my suggestion for good back health was very progressive and thanked me for bringing it to his attention! I was convinced that my new Rolls-Royce office chair, my new policy of taking daily walks at lunchtime, plus cutting back on my partying would change my pain levels.

Of course it didn't.

In 2003 my dear dad, who was only fifty-eight, was dying of kidney cancer, so many of my weekends and early evenings were spent in Beaumont Hospital. It was a very difficult time for everyone in the family and we were all struggling to cope. David and I moved into my parents' house to help support them. I put my increased pain and headaches down to the stress of my working life and the personal difficulty I was having in coming to terms with my dad's prognosis. In hindsight this was probably the catalyst for my decisions that followed. I was still feeling the pain and decided that stress might be a factor. Maybe the source of my pain was in my head? Perhaps it was a reaction to the stress in my life and all the extra work I was doing in Lillie's Bordello? I resolved to make some big changes to my lifestyle.

Around this time, I heard of yet another 'miracle worker' – a Chinese herbalist who had cured all sorts of illness – and thought he would definitely be able to help me. I made an appointment. In hindsight, many of his observations were probably accurate: I was tired, I was over-worked, I was stressed. He also said that my pain was related to candida – I was allergic to yeast. If I stuck to a strict, boring diet I would detoxify my body and feel the benefits, and hopefully wouldn't feel the pain! So instead of enjoying my mother's wonderful Irish Mammy comfort food, I was eating very dull food and taking all sorts of supplements to heal my leaky gut. My herbalist also spoke about my sacral chakra area; this is where we keep stress, he said. Apparently I didn't like where I was 'sitting' in life.

I took all this very seriously. Where was I 'sitting' in life? I started to ask myself if I was really happy at work. Was I really happy in my relationship? Was I really happy with myself? I decided to see a counsellor and we worked through some issues I was having at the time. This helped a lot and I would say I am a much better person today for doing those sessions, but unfortunately it didn't resolve the pain or uncover any deep reason for having it. However, the counselling did help me accept that the pain was a physical thing that was happening in my body, so at least I wasn't imagining it. It was nice to know I wasn't mad after all; it was real and it was there!

David and I spent over a year living with my parents and during this time I had a great opportunity to really look at my life. I questioned every aspect of my life and decided only to do things that I really loved doing. When you watch a parent die slowly from a crippling disease, your own life flashes in front of you. It was during this time that I decided to do something for fun, so I began to study for my Speech and Drama Associate of the London College of Music (ALCM) teaching diploma. It was a welcome escape from work and from the hospital during this difficult time; I desperately needed a distraction from the physical and emotional pain that seemed to consume my every thought.

28th February 2005

Dad is back in hospital. We have been told officially they can't cure the cancer, it has spread far and wide. I am feeling so sad. Watching him deteriorate is beyond painful. I am not sure I know how to deal with it. I know I should write down how I am feeling now instead of worrying about what is inevitable and going to happen soon. I have no energy, I want to retreat into myself and be alone. I need to be strong for Mam. Maria and the kids are over this weekend, Dad will be pleased. Please angels help me deal with this, it's so hard. Thank you. x

After almost two years of battling cancer my father passed away in Beaumont Hospital on 23 April 2005, surrounded by all his children and with my mother holding his hand. It was, in all probability, the worst day of my life. As I looked out of the window, all I could see was tree after tree of beautiful cherry blossoms in full bloom.

I took a brief period off work to grieve and help my mam adjust to life without Dad. However, when I returned to the busy world of post-production I felt different. Was the combination of stress, grief, pain and sadness I was feeling just too much? I confided in a friend and colleague about how I was feeling, and they recommended that I make an appointment with a highly regarded GP. So I did, and I also wrote out a list of things to mention to her. I wanted to clearly explain about my history of mysterious body pain, about my tiredness, how little tasks were becoming difficult and how I had trouble sleeping.

After much discussion, the doctor told me that my symptoms must be related to stress and grief, and before I knew it I was taking my first anti-depressant tablet. Those tablets just floored me. I felt as though I was in an emotional straitjacket. My hands were tied, my senses were tied and my feelings were tied. I was just numb to life and, in a way, numb to the pain. I stayed on those tablets for three months and those months are a blur. I can't remember things that happened; often people remind me of events from that time, but I was on autopilot and have no memory of what they are describing.

I do know that during this time I passed my ALCM teaching diploma with flying colours and took this as a sign that maybe I should consider a change in career, so, although I had spent many happy years in a job I loved and was well suited to, I tendered my resignation. It was a really tough decision, but I felt I needed to close that chapter of my life and try to get control and some sense of understanding of what was going on inside my body and brain.

I know this was a very worrying time for David and luckily he could see that my problems wouldn't be resolved by taking anti-depressants. With his support I stopped taking them and started to really look at my lifestyle again. But the same question still confronted me. What was causing this pain?

5

Searching for Answers

By August 2005 I had resigned from Windmill Lane and also my hostessing job in Lillie's. I left behind a circle of close work friends and, as I wasn't based in the city, I couldn't just meet them after work for a glass of wine and a chat, or a lunchtime coffee catch-up. The isolation this caused was compounded by the fact that David and I had finally finished building our new house. It was in a new area on the other side of the city from where I was born and had been living, so I didn't know anyone. My world, which had been buzzing with things to do and people to see, was suddenly very small. Some days I would only see David and maybe the postman. My new, trusted friend was my adorable little puppy, Dash, who kept me sane and loved during that awful, lonely and confusing time.

The pace of my life had dramatically changed, but slowly, in September of that year, I began working a few hours a week, doing part-time voice-over continuity work for TV3. I also made use of my Speech and Drama teaching diploma, teaching in Betty Ann Norton's drama school in Dún Laoghaire on Saturdays and covering maternity leave for a speech and drama teacher in a local school. I had much more free time than ever before and, in sharp contrast to the busy Windmill Lane days, my stress levels were zero. I wasn't desk-bound any more, either. Now my work was mostly done standing up and I did notice a difference in the pain. Yet it remained a constant companion, like my shadow, an ever-present reminder that, despite everything I was doing, it was still there.

In fact, as time passed, I seemed to be becoming more and more consumed by the pain. Perhaps I was also getting a little paranoid – I felt embarrassed and ashamed for even feeling it. In my head I had no legitimate cause or reason for this daily pain. Maybe because I had seen not only my father, but many of my mum's sisters – one as young as thirty-nine – die of cancer, I began to wonder if I had a very serious disease and was getting worse, maybe even dying, and yet nobody seemed to be taking it seriously.

If pain is the body's defence mechanism, my body was trying to tell me that something was wrong and no one seemed to know what it was. Worse still, I felt it was taking control of my life. I was in a constant low, sad state and was scared that I would end up alone, with only Dash for company! Sometimes I actually wanted to be alone, because every day David would ask me what I had done with my time and, really, I wasn't doing an awful lot in comparison to the old me.

The pain also affected me at night, so I was having trouble sleeping. Yet I was spending more and more time in bed; I didn't feel anyone believed me about my pain and I felt hopeless. No matter what I said or did, people judged me or had an opinion about what was wrong with me. It was a mess and I was a mess, but of course I couldn't see that and no one could really talk to me because I was so sensitive about it. Something had to change. It was time for another family intervention!

Apart from the constant worry about pain, life was really good for me and David. In 2006 David surprised me with a trip to Dubai and proposed in the Burj Al Arab. Planning for the wedding was a great distraction and, after nine years together, we married in the magical, romantic city of Venice the following year. Naturally, after the wedding, lots of well-meaning friends and family hinted at the prospect of babies and starting a family, and it was one such conversation that led me to reveal my fears about the constant pain.

In the summer of 2007 I visited my eldest sister, Lavinia, who was living in the UK. Even though we didn't see each other very often, she recognised that something was wrong. I revealed my concerns about the pain, and she believed me when I told her that I genuinely felt something was seriously wrong with me. She asked her husband, a doctor, to arrange for me to get a full MRI scan on my lower lumbar area to see if there was any underlying reason for the mysterious pain.

A few weeks later David and I travelled to the UK hoping to get answers. After a day catching up with family we went to the Spire Alexandra Hospital in Kent for my scan. The loud noise of the scanning machine brought me right back to the spring morning in 2003 when I drove my dad to his first scan in the Blackrock Clinic in Dublin. He had described to me the distinctive loud sound of the machinery and how he was strapped onto the bed before it went slowly into the tunnel. We laughed together afterwards, as he said to me, 'Thank God it wasn't your mother going into the MRI as her claustrophobia would certainly have sent her over the edge of fear and anxiety.' During my own scan I felt a huge sadness remembering my dad, and how vibrant and full of life he was that morning. We never expected his scan to show up anything serious or life-threatening, as he had looked perfectly healthy. Anyone looking at him wouldn't have guessed (as we hadn't) that within eighteen months he would be dead. A desperate sense of fear was creeping over me.

Probably one of the hardest things to deal with when you have chronic pain or a mysterious pain is the feeling that no one believes you. Then you can start to doubt yourself too. I felt there was something genuinely wrong with me. I knew I wasn't imagining it as the pain was so real, but no one else could detect it or find its source and no GP I had seen before had even suggested an MRI. I was thinking, 'I'm a healthy young woman – why am I feeling this pain? Please, please, please let something show up on this scan, please God let me find some answers, and please, make someone believe me and help me get rid of this pain for ever!'

Back in Ireland I couldn't wait to get the results. The call came just as I was about to get into my car in the TV3 car park. My brother-in-law Graeme said that the scan had detected small disc osteophytes at L3/4, L4/5 and L5/S1, causing spinal stenosis, which he described as narrowing and displacement of nerve roots that puts pressure on the spinal cord and nerves which can cause pain. I seemed to be worse on my left-hand side. Spinal stenosis is most common in people over fifty, so, being in my twenties, this was an unexpected diagnosis to get my head around. Graeme made a joke about me getting old and that all the partying had finally caught up with me. He is a very chilled type of person, so we laughed a bit, which settled any concerns that something serious was wrong with me. He said that he would look into pain treatment options and give me a call in a couple of days.

Once again I had a name to put on the pain. I had a rational reason for it; I could say I had a diagnosis. In my heart I felt that finally someone knew what was wrong with me, that we could now move on and treat this pain, and I would be cured. I felt upbeat and positive about the future; hope is a great thing. The vision of a future alone with Dash was fading. I felt that without the pain, maybe I could return to Windmill Lane. I had been busy with some freelance production jobs, people still wanted to hire me, so maybe I could get my life back. I would be happy again.

Within weeks I had an appointment with a pain specialist in the UK, who suggested an injection into the coccyx area to treat the pain. She seemed very confident that this would be successful. Initially, it did seem to work – I had no pain, I felt like a new person. I celebrated with my sister, we drank champagne – it was a miracle, the doctor had cured me! Immediately I slept better and woke up telling everyone I had had the best night's sleep. It may have been the amount of champagne I had consumed, but I felt really great. I seemed to have more energy and we had even gone out dancing; it was a super, fun weekend.

Sadly, within a few days that small niggle of familiar pain returned, not strongly, but when I felt it, I tried to pretend it wasn't there. I desperately wanted to be cured. I cried alone in the toilet of my sister's house, not wanting to tell David or my family that the pain was back. I'm not sure that I really mentioned it until I was back in Dublin. I suppose I was thinking that it might go away again. And I felt stupid. How could I tell all these people, who had celebrated with me because my pain was gone, that it was back? I prayed I would go to sleep and when I woke up it would be gone. 'Please, just go away,' I thought. 'I will do anything, God, just make it go away. I want to keep celebrating, I want to have all that happy energy. Why is the pain back?'

Once again I felt alone, isolated, unsure of how my body was feeling and blaming myself for having this burden of pain, which now seemed to be consuming not just my life but my family's and, most of all, David's too.

Now that David and I were married, starting a family was something we had discussed, but I was beginning to wonder about the effect my constant pain was having on our marriage. Who would want to be with someone who can't seem to function on a very basic level without being in pain? Maybe I wouldn't be able to have children, and if I could, how would that affect my pain levels? I no longer felt like the fun-loving girl I used to be when

I met David. Everything about my life was very serious, joyless, and I felt really sad inside. I was confused about what I should do next. I didn't feel I could talk to anyone about what and how I was feeling; I felt I had used the word 'pain' too much with my family. I thought I needed to pretend that everything was okay, not just for my sake but for my family and for David. Then again, that made me feel madder and more isolated.

The pain specialist in the UK had suggested to me that I use a TENS machine daily for the pain. We had bought one while over there and I had been using it every day without fail, but while the pain had decreased a little, it was still there. For a couple of weeks after we came back from the UK, I didn't really talk about the pain and I really tried to act as though it wasn't there, but the familiar aching, almost cutting feeling in my lower back and buttocks persisted, despite my best efforts to forget it. I remembered those few wonderful full nights of restful sleep I had enjoyed before the injection had worn off and I felt I would do anything just to be able to sleep like that again. Often I would wake during dreams that I was having electric shocks in my back to find that I had awoken because of the pain.

After weeks of poor sleep and the stress that comes from constant pain – the pain takes over everything – I started to take huge volumes of over-the-counter tablets to dull the pain. I also started to have regular evening glasses of wine, to help with the pain and to knock me out so that I would sleep. At that time the evenings were the hardest for me. David wasn't saying much, but clearly he could see that I was drinking every night and that I was generally not very happy. Then I would berate myself for drinking and stop for a few days, but quickly start again. This became a vicious circle and it clearly wasn't working – if anything I was feeling worse and it wasn't helping my mood or, indeed, the pain.

Eventually, one night, in a semi-drunken state, I locked myself in my bathroom and found myself crying again on another toilet floor. I felt so low. How could I possibly burden people with this when everyone else had serious worries in their lives? My mother was now a widow, still very much grieving for the loss of my dad; David's dad had been diagnosed with prostate cancer, although thankfully his treatment was successful and he was doing very well. I felt that, in some way, I was failing. I was failing to get better and I was constantly thinking about my pain when other people had real reasons to be in pain. I didn't even know what was causing mine. And now a similar pain appeared to be starting in my neck, so I had head and neck pain on and off, as well as aching lower back pain that sometimes would shoot down my legs. As I lay on the floor distraught over the state of my life I was convinced I needed to be in a mental hospital, or else I was actually dying of a rare disease and no one had diagnosed it yet. The alcohol, anxiety, self-pity, pain and self-loathing completely took over and I ended up crying uncontrollably for what seemed like hours. I didn't want to leave the bathroom; I wanted time to freeze so I could just stop moving on with my life. It seemed to me that everyone was getting on with their lives and I was just being held back with this burden of pain.

David knocked on the door. He asked me to open the door and talk. I remember crying out: 'Why would you want to be with me?' I told him I felt lost and needed a miracle.

That night he just hugged me and told me that everything would be okay; we would get through this; there was light at the end of the tunnel. I laughed and said that with my luck it's probably the light from an oncoming train.

Without David's love and support, I really think I would have gone insane.

6

New Doctor, New Hope

In late 2007 I made an appointment with Dr Paul Murphy in the Blackrock Clinic, a pain doctor I hoped might be able to help. Once again, my hopes for a pain-free life were wrapped up in a doctor I had yet to meet. I prayed that he would be able to help me get my life back again.

Constant pain, coupled with the exhaustion from lack of sleep, makes routine activities very labour-intensive. It's very difficult to carry out even the most basic tasks when all you can think about is the burning pain radiating around your body. I hadn't really discussed it with any close friends and really the only people who could see the effect it was having on me were David and my mam.

The meeting with Dr Murphy went really well. He asked a lot of questions. He described the pain in ways that no other doctor had described it to me before, and I felt he believed me. I felt he understood. There were a lot of new words and explanations for why my back might be in pain, but he said that the first step was to try to get the pain under control. He was also very concerned about the broken sleep and really wanted to try to fix that. He seemed to be able to piece together all the bits of information I had given him to create a clearer picture of how I was feeling and coping than even I could articulate. It was clear that he had a huge understanding of chronic pain and empathy with me as a patient. As I sat in his office I felt that maybe, just maybe, a miracle was possible.

Dr Murphy said that we would start with some tablets, see how they worked and go from there. Then, although I was embarrassed as David was there and we hadn't discussed it beforehand, I asked if any of these tablets might affect me getting pregnant. There was a pause, a silence, and then Dr Murphy asked me: 'Are you trying to get pregnant?'

I said, 'No, but ...'

'We need to tackle the pain first. Take this year to sort out the pain and then we can review the situation. I understand absolutely that starting a family is very important and we can aim for that in the future,' he replied.

Although I had probably kept Feminax in business in Ireland for years, I hadn't often had to take prescription tablets, so being instructed to take two different tablets daily was a bit of a shock. When Dr Murphy explained how the tablets worked and why they worked, it was all very new to me. The first one he described as an anti-epileptic or anti-convulsant. It worked by slowing down the signals to the brain that affect pain signals in our nervous system, and he said that there was good evidence that it was very effective against neuropathic pain associated with spinal cord injury. The other, which I would be taking at night, is usually prescribed for depression, but it also seems to be effective for sleep and is widely used against chronic neuropathic pain.

I was a bit worried about the anti-depressant, as I had had a terrible reaction to the one I had taken after my dad had died, but Dr Murphy explained that the dose was very small and really it would only work on the neuropathic pain.

My next question was, 'What *is* chronic neuropathic pain?' I can't remember his answer in detail, but he explained that it is a chronic state of pain: the nerve fibres – the nerves themselves – may be damaged or dysfunctional and can sometimes produce pain signals even when there is no physical pain source. So, for example, long after an injury people may still feel 'nerve' pain at the injured site. I think he may have mentioned phantom limb pain, where people who have had an arm or leg removed still experience pain in the amputated limb. Dr Murphy also mentioned how the sensation of nerve pain would often be as I described it – an aching or burning. The 'creepy-crawly tingling' feeling I had mentioned was, he said, very typical of neuropathic pain.

That really surprised me, as I hadn't really told anyone that it felt like a creepy-crawly tingling feeling, like pins and needles. But that, and even the electric-shock type pain, seemed to be a perfect way of describing it. This was a major 'Aha!' moment for me. Dr Murphy was able to piece together my weird symptoms and understand that it was all linked. At the time I had also been getting an intermittent ache in my right leg. It wasn't really pain, but it was exactly like a creepy-crawling feeling; to me it was just an uncomfortable sensation – it wasn't like the dull ache in my coccyx – but it all seemed to be related!

This was the miracle I had hoped for. At the very least, for the first time ever I was clearly understood and I was believed. I felt relieved. Now I had a new name for my pain and a reason for it. I don't know why this was so important to me, but it was all about having something to blame for my pain and something to call it. It was not visible to the human eye (out of sight, out of mind), but having a name for my pain – neuropathic pain – that sounded official, medical, validated it in some way. I had met a doctor who understood and now when anyone asked, 'What's wrong?' or 'Why are you not coming out?' or 'We didn't see you at that event', I could at least say, 'I have a neuropathic chronic pain condition.' The trouble was, then they might say, 'What exactly is that? How did you get it?'

So once again Google became my friend and I would look up chronic pain and try to understand it as much as possible. If

I didn't understand what was wrong with me, how could anyone else? There were so many different definitions:

> Neuropathic pain, a chronic pain as a result from an injury to the nervous system.

> Neuropathic pain is another term for nerve pain.

> Neuropathic pain can be a complication of conditions which are associated with nerves.

> Neuropathic pain is caused by damage or disease affecting any part of the nervous system involved in bodily feelings often described as 'burning', 'tingling', 'electrical', 'stabbing', or 'pins and needles'.

At the time in a way I felt validated that my 'neuropathic' pain was different to acute normal pain. I was surprised I had never heard the term for this type of pain before and even more shocked to read on my Internet searches just how many hundreds of people of all ages worldwide had the same pain as me! I wasn't alone after all.

As well as having the mental relief of having a name for my condition, the physical symptoms were also relieved. I have to admit the tablets worked much better than my Feminax fix. I suppose the biggest revelation was sleep. I also noticed that the strange, creepy-crawly feeling in my leg was reduced too. Previously I hadn't been sure if this was an actual symptom, as it was a very different sensation to the coccyx pain. In some ways I would often think it was just pins and needles and I knew everyone got those, so I didn't feel it was a legitimate reason to complain. I suppose I just thought pain was normal.

With my mood elevated by my new friend, sleep, I was able to embrace my life again. I was in much better form, in less pain, happy and hopeful for the future. I felt a little like myself again and I wanted to work and socialise again. Things were going really well.

To my surprise, around this time the new head of programming at TV3, Ben Frow, made the decision to use in-vision continuity links. A set was being built and they wanted a male and female duo to make introductions to the shows, rather than using voice-overs as we traditionally did. This change was to start in the new year. I had, by then, been the female voice of the station for three years, hovering below the radar, and that suited me well. I was the daytime voice-over, while Conor Clear was the male voice for the evening peak schedule. We worked on opposite shifts and days so I rarely saw him in work. When it was announced that TV3 was looking for two presenters to audition for the in-vision continuity, I honestly hadn't really considered going for it until a chance meeting with Conor in the corridor. We stopped to chat and I asked him what brought him into TV3 as it wasn't his allocated shift time. He very excitedly told me that he had auditioned for and been offered the job as the male in-vision presenter, and asked if I was going for the female role. It was a funny moment that I often laugh to myself about now. I hadn't gone for the role or even expressed an interest in it, but at the same time I hadn't thought through the prospect of losing my handy voice-over gig. Naturally the 'new female' would get the in-vision continuity role, and probably any other voice demands beyond that, so I would end up without a job. In a very positive tone, Conor said, 'You've been doing the job for three years now; you should at least go for it!'

For the first time in months I felt my drive and ambition return in one big gush of emotion, and poor Conor got the brunt of it. I think he thought I was a little mad as I suddenly said, '*Yes!* I *should* be seen for that job!' with more energy and gusto than he was expecting. I think I may have even started to cry just a little. In my mind, I felt this was taking back control of my life – my pain was under control and my future was bright. Why shouldn't I expect to be seen when I was capable – and more than capable – of doing it?

I got the job. It was probably the best thing that ever happened to me. It was the perfect time for me to be embracing work, and one big advantage was that it was work I could do while standing! No more long hours sitting at a desk. One of the best things about doing the in-vision, which I started in January 2008 and was involved in for the next two years, was that I was working every day with two people who became true, loyal and wonderful friends to myself and David: my best friend and partner in crime, Conor, and our cameraman, producer, director, and the funniest man working in TV, Paul Daniel. If laughter is therapy I certainly got lots of that working with them – we laughed a lot and had fun, and everything was light and easy-going.

My time working with Conor and Paul took me out of a very dark place and brought laughter and fun back into my life. I believe we all meet people for a reason and, in a bizarre twist, Paul's wife and now a dear friend, Enda, suffered from chronic pain from various illnesses. I had never met anyone else with chronic pain. For the first time I had friends who totally understood what I was going through. I truly feel that they were supposed to come into my world, bring a wonderful light into my life and support me on my journey at the time.

The only downside to being in vision on TV is that you can't hide it if you're gaining weight. As the old saying goes, 'Seeing is believing'! When I started filming the in-vision daytime links, I was a pretty standard weight. My weight had remained the same all through my twenties, give or take a few pounds. Like most women,

I had my fat days and 'looser trousers' days, but I never really had a problem with controlling my weight. I was lucky – I could eat a lot and not put on too much weight. But, as the months passed, my new tablets meant I gained weight. I don't have weighing scales at home, so I was probably trying to pretend it wasn't happening, but I couldn't hide from it – it happened literally in full view of the nation. Week by week my weight increased and I actually got very paranoid about it. My excuse was that TV puts on the pounds; it wasn't me putting on weight. Right?

Sometimes viewers would send in texts and comments about certain clothes not being appealing, but once a text came in about me getting very 'stout'. We all laughed at the word 'stout' and at the time I didn't think it bothered me, but it did. When I went home, I googled 'weight gain' and the name of one of my tablets. It was clear that they did cause big weight gain in a short period of time. I started to think about stopping the tablets.

It was a difficult decision: having less pain was wonderful, it was making me happier and my life was so much more fulfilling, but I really didn't like the effects the tablets were having on my body. I never felt full. I was eating all the time and always hungry, so my clothes got bigger and bigger and even bigger. However, I decided the benefits of the pills outweighed the downside and realised I had to make peace with the side effect of weight gain. This was hard, as I felt it became the talk of the office and, maybe because I was on TV every day, people felt that they should help me or advise me. At one point, a senior colleague (who is now a good friend) called myself and Conor into the office to talk through the daytime links. After much skirting around the issue and using hand signals to suggest I was getting a little bigger, he said that some people in the office were going to start a Weight Watchers group and I should join too. I know that he only wanted the best for me, but it wasn't what I wanted to hear at the time. To make matters worse, at that point very few people knew about my pain issues, no one knew I was on medication and so people didn't know I had a medical reason for my weight gain. I felt I had to do something, but I wasn't sure what, and, if I am honest, I started to feel really down about it.

I mentioned the problem to Dr Murphy and he did say that it was a side effect that some people experience. As the tablets were not fully getting rid of all the pain, I was also undergoing various treatments, including branch nerve block injections: a day procedure in St Vincent's Hospital. This procedure temporarily interrupts the pain signal being carried by the medial branch nerves that supply a specific facet joint in the backbone. I had had lots of different procedures to different facet joints; in the early days it was trial and error as we didn't know which facet joints were causing the pain. I also had some rhizotomy procedures: this involves the destruction of the nerves in the facet joints, normally by burning them with radio frequency current. On every visit to the hospital I was routinely weighed and my height was taken and noted in my chart, presumably so that the anaesthetist could work out the correct sedative. My weight was slowly creeping up, higher and higher. I actually got a bit obsessed with my weight gain at each weighing in.

I decided that I had to lose weight. I tried the cabbage soup diet and lost no weight. I may even have gained a pound or two. If anyone's spent a week eating nothing but cabbage soup, then stood on the scales and seen that they've actually gained weight … well, it's not a good day. Yet, apart from the extra weight, I looked really healthy and felt a lot more positive because my pain was so much better. Spanx were my best friend at this point, and still are! I struggled to get them on before I was due to shoot any in-vision links, but after deciding I wasn't going to stop my medication, I became an expert on shape wear and how to disguise the extra pounds.

My life was definitely better, I was very happy with my doctor and I was really hopeful that the various procedures at St Vincent's would get rid of the pain for good. I didn't quite truly grasp the concept of pain management: I fully believed that either the nerve blocks, facet injections, rhizotomies or another magic procedure would sort out the rogue nerve and we would cut it off. I would then come off the tablets and my life would be permanently pain free. I was still not sharing my private world of hospital procedures with anyone – it was very much my secret. I suppose I had decided that I would talk about it only when I was cured.

Looking back, I wasn't really managing as well as I thought. The tablets and procedures were only masking the pain and my expectations weren't really attainable. I wanted to be completely pain free – I was still looking for a miracle cure from my doctor. After each procedure I got progressively more annoyed that we hadn't managed to sort it all out. It seemed to be taking a long time and, to be honest, going into hospital for a day procedure seemed a bit dangerous. It was stressful: after all, no one likes to be in hospital, even as a day case. I worried that putting all those needles into my back couldn't really be okay; maybe they would cause more pain – and sometimes they did. Sometimes I might get a small increase in the pain for a few days before I saw the benefit and, honestly, this scared me.

Ultimately I didn't want to be in hospital, and hiding the fact that I was going in and out of hospital was wearing me out. It was a big juggling act at the time, trying to switch shifts so that I could take the time off to go in for my day procedures, then lying low for the weekend after a hospital visit if I wasn't feeling well enough to see people. And of course, the continuing disappointment of the pain recurring, again and again, was taking its toll on me emotionally. At the time I didn't understand the concept that the various different procedures were just for managing the pain. I wanted it gone for good and that wasn't happening and I had a growing sense of disappointment.

Yet all the while I had to show my happy face to the world. Occasionally there were social occasions – maybe friends' birthdays or work parties – that I felt I really had to attend. I would leave the hospital at the end of the day and have to get ready to go out again in the evening. I felt I was living a lie, that every time I went out it was a reminder of how different I was from everyone else. Living with and managing a chronic condition, and trying to appear 'normal' at the same time, was exhausting.

I realise now that my big problem during this period was that no one knew what I was going through. A lot of people in chronic pain struggle with this; will they or won't they tell people? You are often worried about people's reactions. Will people believe me? Can I face the rejection and heartache of not being believed? For me, I didn't want to be seen as weak and I didn't want pity. So I kept my secret.

On a positive note, though, as far as work was concerned I was very busy. I was working hard, getting out more and being offered more work. During that time I was offered a more permanent role on a radio station for which I had been doing a little bit of work, on and off, for the last two years. It came as quite a surprise when I was offered an opportunity to cover evening links for *Mellow Moments* and a Saturday music show on Sunshine 106.8. I really loved the music and the station. When Sean Ashmore made me the offer, I said, 'I'd really love to take it, but I feel I must be honest with you about something. I'm getting some procedures on my back and I might need to go into hospital occasionally on a Saturday.' It was a big admission for me at the time, as Sean was the first person I had really mentioned it to professionally. I was anxious that I would lose out on this great opportunity, but I felt I needed to be honest, as I didn't want to appear to be unreliable.

There was a moment of silence, then I said, 'I can tell you in advance when I need to take time off – it won't be a last-minute thing.'

More silence.

'Hopefully it will be resolved soon so no more visits will be needed.'

Sean seemed to have a little think. I was certain the job would be gone, but to my surprise when he eventually answered he said, 'Yes, that should be okay, once we can plan cover in advance.'

I was delighted and truly shocked, to be honest. Then he said, 'I saw you the other morning with Conor on the TV, and you looked very chirpy. What's wrong with your back?'

I can't remember exactly what I said; probably the traditional Irish response to everything – 'It's grand.' I explained that I was just getting some procedures, but that it was nothing to worry about, and that was that.

So, by March 2009 I had a weekly radio job at a station I truly loved and I was still working for TV3. To outward appearances I was 'grand'; the tablets and procedures had reduced the pain enormously, which in turn was having a very positive effect on my life. I felt a massive sense of gratitude to my miracle doctor, Dr Murphy, who had helped me get some normality back into my life. It was thanks to him I was working, I was busy, I was out and about, and I did feel a little more like the old me.

However, deep inside I was desperately praying for no pain at all – a reduction wasn't enough for me. I was still 100 per cent convinced that I was just one procedure away from cracking this once and for all. Dr Murphy would find the nerves causing the pain and all would be well, nerve gone, pain gone. For ever!

Of course that wasn't the case and the systematic day procedures continued. After another two or three months I was wiped out, both mentally and physically. I couldn't grasp that the pain wasn't going away and that I still needed the tablets. There seemed to be no end in sight and, because I hadn't told anyone else, myself and David were carrying this health burden by ourselves. I look back now and feel so sorry for him having to deal with me and my constant hospital visits, yet having no one to confide in. We did eventually start to tell close family and friends, but few people really knew.

I have few strong memories from that time of new pain medication and treatments in St Vincent's. I really started to notice how much I was isolating myself from others, largely because I was so wrecked after each procedure. Radio has the benefit of sound without pictures. Nobody could see how dishevelled I was in the studio on a Saturday after my hospital visits. I did still have to do the daytime links in TV3, but since I had confided in Conor and Paul, no explanations were needed. If I wasn't feeling too good, they would often joke with me about 'taking my tablets' and it is amazing what you can hide with a good hair and make-up team! Plus the job itself was very easy: we watched TV, we made some comments, maybe announced a competition or talked about the goings-on in the soaps; it was light-hearted and fun and in a way a little escape from the seriousness of living in pain.

The few other people – close friends and family – who knew about my hospital visits, I tried to avoid. I know that sounds like an odd thing to do, but I realised that they felt my disappointment and it upset them to see what I was going through. But it was also because I simply didn't know what to say when they asked, 'How are you?' or if I was planning a family, or why they hadn't seen me, or 'Are you better now?'

I didn't know what to tell people – I didn't even know the answers myself.

Secretly I was battling to keep my life normal, if you could call that normal. I felt really under pressure with the secret hospital visits. I was determined to put on a brave face, to appear to be in control – I clearly have big control issues! At this time in my life, my pain and body felt out of control. I felt that there was some reason why the pain kept coming back, I just didn't know what that reason was. Plus I couldn't seem to lose weight. Everything seemed beyond my control.

The tablets were having other side effects that I couldn't see at the time. For the first time in my life I seemed to have a low sex drive. I was secretly feeling very insecure about this, and I felt that I was unattractive to David and that's why our sex life was suffering. I blamed myself, my weight; I was constantly berating myself about everything. Yes, my life was busy, but I felt that my work ethic and drive were gone. I wasn't working the long crazy hours I had done in Windmill Lane, nor was I socialising very much in town any more, so something was wrong with me. I just felt like a moaner, constantly going on and on to David about this mysterious pain.

In hindsight I realise that all this was a side effect of the medication. I was new to the drugs and my reactions to them, so I didn't feel I had any right to question my doctor about them. The various different treatments – branch blocks, facet pain injections, rhizotomies – didn't seem to be working fully, so I couldn't go and tell Dr Murphy that I thought the tablets were having other strange effects too. I was beginning to feel a little 'hazy', almost like being in a daze at times. I felt the medication was making my mouth dry, sometimes I felt dizzy, and I had constipation, stomach cramps and mouth ulcers! It was a long list and I was afraid Dr Murphy would just think it was me. And I truly believed, maybe it *was* just me. I also felt that if I said anything I would be branded a hypochondriac. The change in my personality, my weight, our relationship, it was all getting on top of me, and of course the pain remained, a lot less than before but still there! Why?

Then a number of events unfolded close together and brought me to the conclusion that I couldn't go on with my life as it was, forcing me to make some life-changing decisions. The first was a close friend's hen-party.

The Saturday of the party, after one of my day procedures, David collected me from the hospital. On this occasion I had taken the day off from the radio station. I was in getting another block and the advice is to take it easy for twenty-four hours, expect the pain to flare, don't drive or drink alcohol. Here I have to give special mention to Dr Murphy's secretary, Kathryn. She has the patience of a saint and such a caring and lovely manner. I have vented every manner of emotion on the phone to her over the years, from crying with pain and desperation to practically declaring I was cured and felt I could run a marathon. Each week, following a procedure at St Vincent's, Kathryn would call and check up on me with such love and tender care. Whatever my mood, she would assure me that she would check with Dr Murphy and get back to me, and she always did! Thank you, Kathryn. And thank you too to Noelle, the new secretary.

On this particular day I wasn't feeling very strong, but I didn't want to miss the hen-party that evening, so I told myself I'd be fine to celebrate this wonderful occasion. On the drive home from the hospital I felt I should really confide to my friend Suzie that I wasn't coping very well, but then I thought, 'I don't want to ruin her night, that's not fair.' So, despite feeling pretty terrible, I convinced David to drive me down to the party for a few hours. It was a fair distance out of Dublin and a long drive. I wanted to be there for Suzie, but I knew I couldn't stay over, so I talked David into not only dropping me down, but driving home and then back again to collect me afterwards. The man has some patience!

It was an amazing evening with wonderful friends, but sadly I needed to leave early. I was so upset and angry that once again pain had spoiled another evening that I cried in the car, mostly silently, for most of the trip home. I kept thinking that this should have been a joyous, fun-filled occasion, and that I desperately wanted to feel part of the gang, dance around, have fun, celebrate, but I was just consumed with pain. On top of that I hadn't really explained to the people there why I was leaving early, so I felt really guilty that I wasn't being a good friend, or that others might judge me as not being a good friend.

Yet another night of cursing this pain I was feeling and asking myself, 'Why? Why? Why? Somebody please tell me why my body is in pain. Why can't I get well, feel better, get rid of this non-stop pain?'

The next big hurdle for me was Suzie's wedding. It was a two-day event and I felt I needed to explain my situation to her and how desperate I was. I called her and explained why I had left the hen-party early. I was honest for the first time about just how low I felt, how much pain I was in and how I felt ashamed of it. Sitting for any length of time was agony, and the thought of having to make the journey to the wedding by car (the venue was a few hours outside Dublin) was unbearable.

Suzie's reaction showed me that I really should have told my friends sooner. She totally supported me and, as David's and my cars were both two-seaters, she even suggested we borrow a larger, more comfortable car to drive to the wedding. In the end we rented a car, which meant that I could lie down in the back seat for the journey. The wedding was wonderful, although I still couldn't fully enjoy it because of my mental state and the pain.

Another social event that unfolded soon afterwards would bring an end to my hospital procedures. I had committed to go to a charity lunch, and I brought my mother as my 'plus one', as she knew what I was dealing with at the time. I was a little sensitive and still upset that I had been going to hospital regularly for 'all these procedures' and 'taking all these tablets' and that, even though the daily pain was terrifically reduced, I was still experiencing pain. Pain reduction wasn't good enough: all I wanted was to get rid of it. That was my goal and the target I felt we had to achieve.

Getting ready for the charity lunch, I should have known that my mood was too low. I really shouldn't have gone. When I had committed to go to the event I had been feeling okay and keen to support a worthy charity. I had interviewed the charity about the event on the radio, and I wanted to help and get involved. Sadly, as often happens, when the day arrived I was experiencing a bit of a pain flare-up. Because of a recent procedure my pain had got worse; it was common for it to get worse before it got better. At the time, though, I just felt more pain, more stress, and gloomy that I really couldn't see any end in sight. So before I even tried on a dress to wear I was down in the dumps.

Then I discovered that none of my dresses fitted me any longer. The dress I had in mind I had last worn perhaps a year before. When I tried it on it was clear I had put on weight, so I moaned to my mam, 'I have nothing to wear!' The Spanx came out and I managed to squeeze into something. Feeling very fat and bloated, I went to the event.

The last thing I needed was someone to point out to me that I had put on a lot of weight. I was pretty miserable on the inside but desperately trying to stay upbeat. I was keeping myself to myself – not my usual sociable self. I was getting through the lunch making small talk and all the time thinking, 'It's almost over, I can head off soon.' Then I went to the bathroom and while I was in the queue, someone who knew me and my family very well declared in a very loud voice, 'Look at you! You look blooming … have you any news?'

I wanted the floor to open so I could just sink into the ground and vanish. I wasn't quick enough with a response, and she obviously didn't recognise the horror on my face. It was a ladies' lunch, so the toilets were packed and everyone had had a few glasses of wine. Given the circumstances, and perhaps having had a little too much to drink, this woman lost all tact and went on, 'Well? Am I right?' Then she said something about a little addition to the family. I felt people staring at me, and I think someone said, 'Is that the girl off the telly?' I almost burst into tears. Everyone was looking at me, at my stomach, waiting for me to answer.

Eyeing the cubicles and willing the door to open I tried to laugh off the conversation, wondering if I should just run out of the bathroom altogether. I felt I had to respond, so I said something like, 'It's not on the cards for us at the moment, I don't think it's the right time just now.' Thinking to myself, 'Please stop talking to me,' I tried to say that I just wanted to use the mirror and moved out of the queue, away from my inquisitive family friend. But, to my horror, she insisted on continuing the questions. Now she moved on to why I wasn't pregnant and suggested that I was obsessed with my career and that I was forgoing a family!

She had no idea just how wrong she was.

Stupidly, I tried to justify my situation by quietly explaining that I was taking medication for my back and really it wouldn't be wise to be thinking that way at the moment. I think after a few glasses of wine she probably wasn't aware of how loudly she was speaking when she repeated what I had just said quietly to her: 'I have a bad back and it's not a good time for children right now.' It clearly struck a chord with her as she declared to the packed room: 'A bad back! Are you for real? I have a bad back! Let me tell you, when you go through childbirth, you'll know all about a bad back!'

And the final blow: 'Andrea! You really need to get over yourself!'

What happened next was a disaster. I should have just walked away. But no, I got angry! I explained my situation to her, telling her about all my tablets, the weight gain, the hospital visits, having a problem with my 'nerve endings'. I can't even remember all of what I said, but it was evidently interpreted by some people there that I was some kind of basket case, so into my career that I didn't want children; that I was using a bad back as an excuse and taking lots of tablets because I had a problem with my 'nerves'. That little tale seemed to gather momentum, because by the time the Chinese whispers came back to me I had apparently had a nervous breakdown and was addicted to tablets!

I can laugh about that story now. It was many years ago. But I recall that day so well. I felt so low, I felt I had to justify my situation, my pain. When I got home, I cried tears of uncertainty, once again asking myself if the pain was real. Maybe everyone has back pain. Why am I taking these tablets, getting these procedures? How could I be a mother? The woman at the lunch was right. How could I deliver a baby? How could I go through the pain of childbirth if I couldn't manage 'back pain'?

Then I wondered, what sort of a person does she think I am? She knows my family, my upbringing. We are all so close as a family and anyone who knows me would know that family has always been very important to me. Of course I really wanted a child, why would she think I was so selfish and only into my career?

Ironically, that television career would come to an end shortly afterwards, in late 2009. Although Conor and I were still on air, there were lots of changes to the daytime schedule in the new year, including a brand-new morning show. A decision had already been made that, after two years, the in-vision continuity was ending at the beginning of the year and it would be back to off-screen voice-overs. So the whole idea of my being a hard-nosed, career-hungry workaholic couldn't have been further from the truth. My real career had been in production, a world of high demands and even higher budgets, where little mistakes cost a lot of money; so being on screen doing a few little links wasn't exactly a high-powered, high-pressure career.

At the time perhaps I still felt a little sadness for the job I had left behind. I hadn't really thought that people would perceive me as 'doing well' in my career by doing the in-vision continuity. It was a fun job, but after that lunch I felt that a number of things in my life had to change: how I lived my life, how I dealt with the pain and the work I was doing. I had to be honest with myself and admit that, after more than a year, I was at a point where I really felt I couldn't do the constant day procedures, the tablets, the secrecy any longer.

At home after the lunch I probably had another bottle of wine, and before I knew it I was in a very familiar place, yet again crying in desperation, praying, 'Please help me. Please, God, help me.' Then there was a knock on the door. I was pretty sure it wasn't God – but David was there again, as he always is. He said, 'Let's go to bed. We can make an appointment with Dr Murphy tomorrow and we can discuss other options.'

Pain-*free* Life

From: Andrea Hayes

To: pmurphy.painspecialist

Sent: Monday, 28 September 2009, 20:58:48

Subject: update

Hi Kathryn,

I just wanted to pass on an update to Dr Murphy following the injection.

Sadly I didn't feel any great pain relief, in fact I am getting a lot of breakthrough pain, so I feel like I am taking over my daily allocated tablets to manage it. I can't seem to get the pain to go completely which is very draining; it's a lot worse when I have to sit down for any period of time.

I spoke to Dr Murphy about the pain management course, maybe we can investigate this further. I am desperate to get some sort of way to manage this pain and hopefully try to get it to go long term; whatever Dr Murphy feels is the best route to go from here I am happy to go along with that.

I am so sorry I don't have positive feedback following the injection.

As always thank you for all your help, I look forward to hearing from you soon.

Kind regards,
Andrea

7

Pain Management Course

Life was certainly changing pretty fast and my biggest lesson was still to come. Following the email, we made an appointment with Dr Murphy. When I again brought up my desire to start a family, he was very understanding and supportive. He had just had a daughter himself, and he reassured myself and David that he would offer every support. He said that an in-house pain management course would be a good option, as it might help me reassess my lifestyle and take a positive approach to dealing with the pain in the future.

The disappointment of the failed procedures, and maybe the effects of the medication, seemed to have taken its toll on me. Once again, I didn't want to socialise, and when I did go out, I would often end up feeling really low afterwards, partly because I didn't feel like everyone else and, I now realise, because the pain can get worse after a night out – though at the time I hadn't realised that.

I had a few weeks to wait before I would be placed on the pain management course, and before then they needed to make sure I was a suitable candidate. As for work, I began to think that if I was going to stay in TV and in front of the camera, I should at least work on programmes I felt I could relate to.

I had heard that TV3 wanted to do a pet and vet show, and the idea of doing a weekly report on the show about animal welfare and cruelty to animals appealed to me. I was unsure if I was in the running, so I felt I had to pitch myself just to be seen for the audition. Luckily I knew the producer and I asked him, very nicely, to give me a screen test for *Animal A&E*. I explained that I was passionate about highlighting the plight of mistreated animals in Ireland, and, if I am very honest, I wanted to shine a light on the pain they suffered in silence. I felt these animals needed a voice, that someone should expose what was happening to these defenceless creatures.

I was delighted when I got the job. At first I did short reports for the show, which was built around the vet side of things. Luckily I was able to self-produce the pieces and I was excited about the new year at my work and going around the country to see the ISPCA at their work. In time the animal welfare side of the show grew to become the main feature. The series went on to be a huge ratings winner and was shown across Europe on the Discovery Channel and on Channel 5 in the UK.

While I was waiting to be assessed for the pain management course, I had decided to make up my own rules for my medication. I wasn't taking the tablets as recommended, I was very withdrawn and I was drinking almost every night, maybe a half a bottle of wine at first – the wine was really my painkiller. This wasn't a good idea, of course, but it's very easy to get into the bad habit of drinking to help your mind switch off from what is really going on. Half a bottle became a bottle most evenings.

During those 'wine nights' I was becoming obsessed with looking up pain and other people's experience of pain on the Internet. I found out through my Internet trawling that, more often than not, mysterious severe pain meant you had cancer. So I became very anxious and worried again, probably partly a side effect from taking my tablets erratically, but at the time all I could think of was that not only had cancer been very prevalent on my mother's side of the family, but my dad had died of cancer and another relation on my dad's side had also recently died of cancer.

I went into panic mode. The more I searched, the more worried I became. I felt concerned that Dr Murphy might have missed something, and once again I started to believe that somewhere inside me a serious undiagnosed disease was getting worse and that I could be dying. My mind raced from cancer to the complete removal of my coccyx. In one of my late-night searches, I had read about someone in America who had had their coccyx removed and they had had no more pain. I seriously considered it. Yes, it seemed drastic, but if it would stop the pain I felt I could handle it.

Then I thought that maybe one of the new doctors I was going to meet on the pain management course could diagnose whatever it was that had been overlooked and that whatever it was – this thing we hadn't discovered – would be removed and then all would be well. I became very optimistic and confident that after the pain management course I would be fixed and pain free, and I planned being able to go snowboarding again, being able to get back to the gym – which I certainly needed after all the weight I had put on in the last year. Dr Murphy wasn't so sure. He thought my pain wasn't ever going to go away.

I believed at this point that my life was simply on pause. In a few weeks, after the assessment and placement on the three-week pain management course, it would resume. I would be able to achieve all my goals, the main one being to start a family. Being on medication, despite my recent erratic behaviour in taking it, still meant that pregnancy wasn't an option, plus the burden on my lower back of my extra weight didn't help, and a half or full bottle of wine a night isn't good for an already expanding waistline.

In November 2009 I had a number of appointments to meet some of the pain management team, as I needed to be assessed for my suitability to take part. This included a physical in a gym. That was the first big shocker. The gym was on the second floor in the hospital – whoever heard of a gym in a hospital? When I turned up, I started to explain that I had serious constant pain and that doing exercise in the gym would make it worse. It was as though the instructor didn't even hear me. The assessment was going ahead, come what may.

I also spoke to a clinical physiologist – I think I shed a silent single tear when I was explaining to her how the constant pain was affecting me – and finally I met an occupational therapist, who discussed my daily routine and work demands. I was struck by how much empathy they seemed to have for what life was like for someone with chronic pain. I felt very comfortable chatting to them and they seemed genuinely pleasant and understanding. Thankfully I was accepted for the course and my hope was that this was finally the answer to my prayers and there would be light and hope at the end of the three weeks.

I began my course in St Vincent's in January 2010. It was a particularly cold Monday morning, and the participants had to meet in a building outside the main hospital; I remember the waiting room felt so frosty I could see my breath as I sat down and got myself settled. After a short while a number of names were called out and we were all brought over to the main hospital to a much cosier room. As I looked around at the other ten members of the group my first reaction was that I could be the youngest. In fact I wondered if I was in the right group, as some of the people had canes and others looked much worse off than me. We sat around, introduced ourselves and explained why we were there. Each person's story was different. I found it fascinating. I would never have known to look at many of them that they were in constant pain. I thought to myself: 'This is going to be tough.'

One of the women had been on the course before and said that she wanted to get back to doing the routine and pacing. She had suffered breast cancer and after her operation she was left in chronic pain from the scar tissue. Though she had survived the cancer many years ago, she was still suffering chronic pain every day. I felt drawn to her and to her story, and over coffee I had a chat with her. She told me that the constant pain was worse than the cancer. At the time that seemed unbelievable. I wondered privately if the doctors had messed up, made some medical error when they operated; I just couldn't get my head around someone being left in permanent pain after the cancer had gone.

We started the first day with some meditation, then there was a talk from a doctor, followed by a coffee break. Then there was some occupational therapy. During this time we looked at all aspects of our lives and how we could make it easier to live and cope with pain better. A word I learned in that first class was 'pacing'; little did I appreciate the massive importance this word would have on my pain management programme. It became almost like breathing for me – that is how important it is in the daily management of chronic pain. However, the exact meaning of 'pacing' varies depending on the person.

Pacing is an active self-management strategy whereby individuals learn to balance time spent on activity and rest for the purpose of achieving increased function and participation in meaningful activities. Our occupational therapist drew a diagram to explain the common yo-yoing pain cycles that chronic pain patients regularly go through. Everyone could identify with the idea of pushing through to finish a task or attend a social event, only to crash and burn and be left with a flare-up of pain for a number of days or even weeks afterwards. And depression can commonly go hand in hand with pain. The therapist explained that we would learn pacing techniques that would help us do things in our lives in a different way. From now on we would plan to do tasks or daily chores in a different way: look at the activity; break down what needed to be done; do it for a period of time; and schedule in rest time. She explained that we needed to stop the activity before the pain and fatigue made us stop. She also said that our thoughts and psychological factors play a significant part in the pain cycle and that the psychologist would look in more detail at our unhelpful automatic thoughts and introduce mindfulness. In essence this multi-disciplinary approach to pain would bring many elements together for us and at the end of the three weeks we would be able to manage the pain better and we would learn to break the cycle of pain. For the first week, though, we were encouraged to monitor our activities and look at the effect they might have on our pain. Could we identify our own patterns? Each day we should write in our pain diary. That day I started my pain journal and continue to use it to this day.

Lunch was a welcome distraction and it was really good to get to know the rest of the patients. We seemed to just get on with each other. In the afternoon we had a session in the gym and this was very difficult for me. Usually I didn't go anywhere near a gym as I felt it made me worse. We had been warned about 'fear avoidance' on the first day – another new phrase that would have a significant impact on my pain journey. Often patients with chronic pain avoid movements and activities that they believe will provoke pain. This leads to disengagement from meaningful activities and often to depression and greater disability. The fear of pain can have a greater impact than the pain itself.

I knew that I avoided certain things out of the fear that I would be in more pain afterwards. One of those things was going to the gym and I found myself wondering whether our physiotherapist, who was now waxing lyrical about the daily exercise routine we would all be participating in, had lost touch with reality. I remember thinking, 'I'm not doing all these circuits! Is she mad?' Luckily I wasn't the only one: someone else raised their hand and said, 'Sorry, I genuinely can't use the bike as I have debilitating leg pain.' It didn't take long for a chorus of complaints to rise from the rest of us about the pain that would prevent us from using the various machines too. For me it was the bike – my coccyx pain would prevent me from sitting on the saddle. Very calmly, our physiotherapist said that this was 'fear avoidance'. She stressed that doing daily exercise and, more importantly, stretching would really help our physical and mental well-being.

By the end of the day we had all done three minutes on each circuit, although I must admit I avoided the two bikes – I stuck to walking or the cross trainer and floor work. We were all shocked when we realised we would be working out in a gym every day, but it was a gym in the hospital so if anything happened at least we were in the perfect place to get help.

In addition to that we had a daily walk down to the beach and along the seafront. The rule was that we couldn't talk about the pain during this time – it was a time out from pain. So in our little groups we spoke about our lives, about the weather – too hot, too cold, very changeable, very close – which seemed to bring us full circle back to pain: 'My pain is worse when it's cold', 'I find I don't sleep when it's hot at night.' So even though we tried not to discuss pain, it did slip into conversations. But it was just amazing to talk to other people who understood a life in pain. Our understanding of each other was terrific and a lot of us were on the same tablets, we had similar descriptions of the pain, we understood each other's flare-ups, and that for me was the biggest revelation on that first day. I felt safe and part of a like-minded group, despite our differences in age and lifestyle.

On that first day I went home exhausted and my pain was a

bit up on normal days, but I was able to tell my husband that I'd been in a gym and that I would be going to the gym every day for the next three weeks!

Another big topic at home that evening was the 'family day'. On the pain management course they recommended that in the final week we invite our spouses and families in for a day, so that they could chat to the doctors and see what we had been doing. I can see why this was such an important part of the course: the person with chronic pain is not the only person whose life changes. Very often the partner or parent of the patient has to deal with how their life has changed too, but no one really focuses on them. I think acknowledging that things also change for them is the first step; it opens up the communication channels. It was of huge benefit to me and to David and it helped us to have more compassion for each other.

I didn't realise that first night, when I asked David to make time for the family day, just how profound it would be. I feel very blessed to have a supportive family around me. Not only did David come in to support me, my mother came too; and on my second pain management course my mother-in-law, Mary, came to the family day. I have no doubt that it was helpful for everyone. It certainly helped me. The families had time alone with the doctors to address any concerns or questions they might have, or their own feelings about the changes in their loved one or in the family dynamic. It was an open platform where they could freely discuss these issues in a loving but honest, straightforward way.

25th January 2010

Dear Diary,

Finished my first day in St Vincent's PMC. It was very interesting. I am exhausted though. I am glad I drove in, parking is going to be expensive but it is easier than trying to find parking on the road and worrying about the meter. I was actually really nervous. As we waited to be admitted I found myself looking around at everyone asking are they on the course? Some don't look like they have chronic pain. Have I made the right decision? I think without question I did. The people are all lovely, really connected with some of them today. Not sure what tomorrow will bring but I am open to everything. On a positive we get coffee and delicious hot fresh scones at 11 and for lunch we go to a staff canteen where the food is actually really good. SO thankfully we will be in a gym every day because I think by the end of the 3 weeks I will have put on a few pounds. Hoping I sleep well tonight, I ran out of one of my tablets, can't believe it happened, so I will need to get to a chemist tomorrow. A x

8

The Day Everything Changed

The second day of that course will be imprinted on my mind for ever, because it was on that day I came to a huge realisation. That was the first day I looked at pain and considered it as a long-term part of my life. I still cry now thinking about that day and writing about it.

I was a little exhausted after the first day, but excited too. The first class of the day was relaxation. As it happened the relaxation CD that we were due to listen to wasn't available. So instead, we talked about the importance of making time for relaxation in our new daily routine.

Next up was psychology and we talked about unhelpful automatic thoughts and introducing mindfulness. I also learned another new phrase for the first time. Cognitive behavioural therapy (CBT) helps you to understand the links between what you think, how you feel and what you do in relation to pain. Many of the tools provided by CBT are very helpful when dealing with pain. There was a lot to take in, and I wanted to explore CBT more, but the class was over too soon; we all had lots of questions and everyone had different topics they wanted to talk about. We were told that later in the day another doctor would come to talk more about the pain and what was going on in our brains and bodies.

Towards the end of the day, everyone was feeling a little overwhelmed by all the new information we were taking in and all the exercise and activity we had been doing. But I was really looking forward to the last lecture of the day by the pain specialist. Again, it was all new information and I was finding it all fascinating. The doctor said he was going to explain the pathways of pain. It seemed very complex and there was a lot to take in, but he tried to simplify it for us. I can still remember him explaining how the dorsal horn of the spinal cord works like a sorting office; it sends signals to the higher parts of the brain (via ascending pathways), and that's where we perceive pain. With the help of a diagram, he explained that with chronic pain the sorting system in the brain often goes wrong and this can lead to changes in how pain messages are processed. He then described how a 'pain gate' can be left open after the original reason for the pain has passed, so that the body still feels pain.

Trying to digest this information was really difficult. I raised my hand and asked: 'When we will we get an accurate diagnosis of our pain so we can address the problem?' Looking back now, I was so naive. In my ignorance I genuinely felt that this was the next step to getting an accurate diagnosis of my mysterious pain problem. I was on a pain management course but I still believed I was there to schedule getting my coccyx bone removed and that this would take away my pain. After all, it was three weeks in hospital, so I had big expectations, all, on reflection, completely unrealistic.

Although the doctor wasn't familiar with my personal medical history, he said: 'You have chronic neuropathic pain. You will always have this pain.'

It still didn't register with me.

I wanted him to clarify this, so I said something like, 'Pain tells the body something is wrong, so all I need to discover is where there is something wrong and sort that out – or in my case take my coccyx out, as that's the location of a lot of my pain. If I can take it out, then logic would suggest the pain will go.'

He looked directly at me and said, 'In your case pain isn't a symptom. It's a disease in its own right.'

He went on to explain that we have this pain because our nerves are misfiring, and he explained more about pain and how changes occur in the nerves and at the cellular level in the body. The normal transmission and modulation processes change, giving rise to unchecked pain. This is known as 'wind-up' – the nerve fibres transmitting the painful signals to the brain become trained to deliver better signals. I don't even know if I'm explaining it correctly because by this point I had gone into a daze. I felt the doctor didn't truly understand, so one last time I raised my hand and said: 'Sorry, can I just ask, if I have chronic pain and there is no logical reason for it, how can I get rid of the pain? People can't live with this pain all their lives. I just haven't been correctly diagnosed yet.'

In a very friendly, but matter-of-fact, way he said, 'Many people live with pain every day. I imagine everyone here is in pain every day; that's why you're all here.'

I looked around and everyone was nodding.

He explained, 'Despite treatment attempts with medication, rest and relaxation, chronic pain may not be effectively relieved. Your doctor has sent you here because things that would usually settle or treat your pain have not been successful for your chronic pain. This is because the problem is with the pain system, rather than being located in any specific part of the body. We are here to help you live with chronic pain daily and reduce the huge impact on your quality of life. You will learn to help yourself to pace your pain.'

I can't really remember much of what he said next because I was in shock. This pain wasn't going away. I actually felt physically ill, every fibre of my being wanted to reject what I had just been told. I wanted to run away and cry, scream and curse – 'This can't be happening!' As the class finished, the doctor said that we had all taken in a lot of new information today, so we should let it settle in and we would pick it up when he saw us again on Friday.

I remember the next few minutes as though they were in slow motion. I left the class and, in the corridor, I burst out crying uncontrollably, tears rolling down my face. One of the ladies from the course put her arms around me; in fact, I felt so faint she was practically holding me up. She looked at me and said, 'You will get through this, Andrea.'

At that exact spot on the corridor there's a little chapel. It's on the first floor of the hospital, in a very quiet spot close to where our classroom was. I had walked by it the day before but hadn't gone in. Now, I thanked the kind lady and I went into the chapel. I sat alone with my thoughts and prayers. Feeling desperate for guidance, I prayed and prayed for a miracle or at least some understanding so that I could achieve some peace. I knew I had no more energy to fight. If I wasn't going to get rid of this pain, I needed to be able to cope with it.

I prayed until I felt I could accept that pain was part of my life. I knew deep down that I needed to make peace with it, I needed to welcome it and learn to accept it, take control of it and not let it take control of my life. I don't know how long I stayed there but it was late when I got home.

For me the biggest lesson I learned on the pain management course was acceptance. Once you have that knowledge, once you know that it isn't going away, you need to be ready for the tsunami of emotions that will follow.

Wednesday 27th January 2010

Dear Angels, universe and God,

I need to stay positive, visualise everything working out perfectly. I am

Pain-*free* Life

in control. I am happy. I am healthy. I will choose healthy foods, detox my body of harsh toxins like alcohol. Tomorrow is a new day. Please help me stay in a place of positivity. I need to stay strong and not allow my disappointment to overwhelm me. Please God surround me this night and give me a positive attitude when I awake and energy to face what tomorrow brings. Thank you God, please hear my prayer. A x

9

Mixed Emotions

Chronic pain is such a personal experience, and during the weeks that followed I realised just how different chronic pain is from any other medical problem. I came to understand that pain cannot be measured like other medical problems. If you have a broken leg or an infection, your broken leg can be confirmed by an X-ray or your infection by a blood test. Unfortunately, for people like me and millions of others, there is no medical test to measure chronic pain, and to make matters more challenging for us, there is often no concrete evidence or physical explanation for the pain.

For the last decade or so, I had experienced exactly what a great many sufferers do – going from one doctor to the next, searching for explanations and hoping with each appointment that this doctor will be the one to discover what is really going on, what is really causing the pain. Something or somebody has to be able to make sense of this pain and help me!

This process of constantly looking for answers had been my life for the last few years, and it was a long and expensive road. I had travelled around the country, even to other countries, searching for answers. I had had unnecessary treatments and procedures, and in some cases the treatments and advice I had had for the mysterious pain had made me feel worse.

I had kept diaries all my life, writing little bits of trivia to remind myself what was going on in my life, but after the first week on the course and the realisation that I had a chronic long-term pain that wasn't going away, I bought a pink writing pad and I began writing a journal about my pain management journey. I wrote every night, mainly to work through my feelings, and I went through a whole host of emotions over the coming weeks.

Shock

This was my first emotion. I was very shocked when I realised that nobody was going to be able to cure me. Even though I had had the pain for so long, I had been certain that it was treatable and it would eventually go. It was just a case of getting the correct diagnosis; meeting the right doctor to prescribe the right tablets or administer the right procedure and then I would be sorted. So I was in total shock to realise that this wasn't the case.

Was this reaction partly because of how we as a society perceive pain? We are taught from a young age that pain is a warning sign from the body that something isn't right, but with chronic neuropathic pain this theory doesn't hold true and everything you believe about pain is challenged. In all my years of searching for answers I hadn't come across anyone being interviewed on television or radio talking about chronic pain, pain that will be with you every day, for ever. I had met Enda, who understood my situation, but she had a number of medical reasons for her pain.

The shock I felt was coupled with confusion, because in addition to trying to understand the news that this pain isn't going away, you wonder how you are ever going to be able to explain this to people. In truth I didn't fully understand it myself, so how would others respond to it? This pain doesn't have a cause and it's not a symptom of anything in particular. Although in the UK I had been diagnosed with lower back spinal stenosis, was that comparable with the pain I was feeling? Probably half of society have that and it's often asymptomatic. So why do I have so much pain when others who have it don't?

Like most back pain sufferers I had been for scan after scan with nothing of great importance ever showing up, so without any tangible reason for this pain how could I explain it to people? It sounds silly, but that in itself was deeply shocking to me.

Mixed with the shock was an overpowering fear: fear for my future, fear of the pain getting worse, fear of becoming paralysed or incapacitated, fear of the pain spreading like ivy on a tree, fear of becoming wheelchair-bound. These irrational thoughts build and gain momentum, and suddenly your future, your dreams and hopes, seem to be on the point of being cruelly taken from you. David and I had been thinking of starting a family. We had been married for almost two years, and together for over ten years, so it was something we had talked about, but because I was taking so many tablets, and with the issue of increased pain with pregnancy, we had put it on hold in the short term. So it was shocking to think I might never be able to start a family, since I was never going to get rid of this pain.

For a day or two I don't think I really talked to anyone. I was totally numb with shock.

Grief

After the initial shock came the grieving process. I cried and cried and cried for a night and I was thinking, 'Why me? Poor me!' A full-blown pity party can unfold very quickly, everything seems pointless and in many ways you grieve for the life you thought you would have, the life and the future that you feel has been abruptly stolen from you. I was so sad, not only for me, but for David, as I really believed it wouldn't be possible now for us to have children. I was convinced that he had married someone who couldn't start a family with him, and worse still, he had tied himself to someone who was facing a life full of pain, not a normal life.

The previous twelve months had been tough for us and what had kept us going was our shared hope for a solution to the pain. Our life had been on hold and we believed that when we sorted out the pain, we could start living again. A terrible sadness overtook me and I grieved for what I wouldn't be able to offer David as his wife. I believed that nothing I did would ever be enjoyable. If you have to deal with constant, debilitating pain, how can you enjoy life? For me the pain grew even bigger in my mind and everything seemed lost to me. I really felt I had lost a part of me – the carefree, hopeful person who believed anything and everything in this life was possible, that if you could dream it, it could happen. I had believed in miracles, but suddenly I felt I needed to change my whole value and belief system. This pain was here to stay and it would rob me of a happy future. I grieved for days.

Anger
Roll out the anger! I was so annoyed at everyone. I was angry at every doctor who had incorrectly diagnosed my pain. I felt let down by the doctors, the specialists, the whole medical profession. I was angry that no one seemed to care that I was in pain, no one had the answers, no one had a plan B, and now they had me on a course where I was being told to just put up with it! That just wasn't good enough! I was furious because I felt I wasn't being treated with the same urgency as other people who were sick.

I also felt angry with the government – why weren't they investing money and resources in research into how someone can be forced to live every day in pain and no one seems to know why or care why? Were we not worth anything? Other patients weren't judged or treated with doubt or suspicion about their sickness, or questioned as to whether their pain was real or 'as bad as they said'. This was a crime against humanity and no one cared! Was it not a basic human right that people should be able to live pain free? Or at the very least, if they are in pain, shouldn't we want to research why? Or at the very, very least *believe* them?

I wanted to scream across the airwaves, '*Why* isn't anyone taking chronic pain seriously? This is a huge problem and no one is helping people like me who live every day in pain. Yes, *pain*, people! I am in *pain*! Why isn't anyone talking about chronic pain in the media? Why hadn't I heard about this until now? Are we not real? Don't people believe we're in pain? Should we just hide behind closed doors and suffer in silence?'

I am a happy person by nature, but this pain was killing me and nobody seemed to give a shit. I wanted to be carefree, I wanted to plan for a family, to be spontaneous, to hop in the car and drive away for the weekend. Instead I had to weigh up every little action according to whether it would cause me additional pain!

After a few days of holding all the anger inside, I broke my silence. I felt like screaming at anyone who judged me. Poor David faced the brunt of my anger; one day, out of nowhere, I just erupted, screaming and shouting at him. I threw my phone at the wall and then collapsed crying on the floor. I was letting all my anger out and arguing with the person who loved me the most and who was dealing with his own shock at my diagnosis. I remember that night so well and to this day I feel terrible that I argued with David; he hadn't done anything wrong. I just hated myself. Why couldn't I be normal and have normal pain? I was also scared that David was having the same thoughts as I was – that I was not good enough for him.

Helplessness

After my outburst I was spent. I had no more energy to fight the pain, to fight for my right to live a pain-free life. What was the point? People didn't even believe that I was in pain. That's why no one was talking about it – no one believed us. Maybe we were all mad. I must be mad. So, with the anger exhausted, another emotion took centre stage – helplessness. It was the weekend after the second week on the pain management course and I was done. I just wanted to stay in bed, close the curtains and cry. I said to David, 'I don't know what to do. I've tried so hard, I've prayed so much for this pain to go, I've done everything and I don't think I can take this any longer.'

Dark days followed and it was a very deflated, much quieter Andrea who went back into the pain management course, feeling a lot less hopeful and pretty helpless. What with the course and my overall mood, I didn't want to talk to anyone for days. I avoided my family and friends. I felt I was broken. But the support, understanding and friendship of the amazing people I met on that course gave me the strength to believe things would be okay; their stories of survival inspired me and I gained strength from their strength. I'm so thankful to have met them. I also have to mention my beloved dog, Dash, who was always at my side, encouraging me, asking me to bring him for a walk. I was blessed to have him; he kept me positive and he was truly my best friend.

Slowly I regained a more positive outlook. The course was amazing. I can't stress how important the multi-disciplinary approach was. By the end of the course I felt stronger and better able to cope. By then, I suppose I knew my life would never be 'normal', but instead of thinking about what I didn't have, I started to focus on my blessings. In my diary – my new ritual – I tried to write what I was grateful for. This was my first entry: 'Thank you universe, angels and God for my wonderful husband, my supportive family, my dog, my home, my friends, my work, my health!'

It might seem strange, but I *was* genuinely thankful for my health. Going into a hospital every day really grounds you – you realise just how truly lucky you are to be able to walk, drive a car, feed and dress yourself, have all your senses. So my helplessness was replaced with a deep sense of gratitude. I wanted to declare it to the world: 'Thank you. I am truly grateful for everything in my life.' And with the love and support of my husband I knew everything would be okay.

Acceptance

Like everyone on that course, I learned to accept that chronic pain is part of my life and that my life's not going to end because of it. This acceptance has many different layers. As time goes by, I seem to gain a deeper appreciation of exactly what acceptance means.

Initially it was a huge switch for me to accept that the pain wasn't going to go away; it felt like I had such a huge mountain to climb. I needed to go back to basics and look to the future in a completely different way, to reshape my plans to include managing daily pain. I would have to create my own life plan, one that would work for me and included time for a daily pain management programme. I needed to make some major life adjustments.

From the first day of the pain management course, the word 'pace' became a daily factor in everything I did. I had to retrain my mind and every day I had to consciously think of pacing myself in my daily routine. It's vital to make this shift. I was re-evaluating every little daily action I was doing, making conscious efforts to take things in moderation, not putting too much pressure on myself to complete tasks and factoring in rest time. In those early days I made a conscious effort to create balance in my life, medically, emotionally, spiritually and socially.

Taking control of one's life in every area has to be an active choice; it doesn't just fall into place. For me it was a case of taking a life inventory, really evaluating my life. I almost treated it as a job. I had to really think about what 'wellness' meant for me. Traditionally, 'wellness' means the opposite of illness and the absence of pain or disease. So I needed to accept that I wanted to create a sense of wellness in my life, to minimise pain and stress. My wellness journey was about living the best possible life I could, while accepting pain as part of that. It wasn't easy, and it took a lot of soul-searching and time to really change how I had been living my life. Every day I would constantly ask myself, 'Will this add to my wellness? Is this good for me? Why am I doing this?'

It was a massive shift. I had to address certain things that needed to change in my life. I started at home. I went through each room and tried to minimise any bending or lifting; anything I used daily was placed conveniently. This proved to be a costly exercise. I realised that so many things in my daily life were adding to my pain and discomfort, so they had to be changed: our bed, the dishwasher, table and chairs and so on. Probably the biggest change was my car; the driving seat needed to be higher and I tried out many different cars to find one where the driving position felt right. Not everything could happen immediately, but basic little things, like rearranging cupboards so that essential items I use daily were conveniently located, really helped me. Often it's the routine things we do that can cause or increase pain and daily wear and tear, and these changes made a real difference to my comfort levels.

I started to reassess the patterns I had been following not just at home, but in every area of my life. I learned to use a great word that I hadn't been using nearly as often as I should: 'No'. I started to say no to social events or work that didn't suit me any more. I also began to say to people, 'Leave that with me. I'll do my best to go, but I can't promise I'll be able to.' I changed my internal dialogue from, 'Andrea, you *should* do this' to 'Andrea, you *could* do this'. Replacing *should* with *could* takes the pressure off. We all have a choice, and I began choosing my wellness over everything else. But while I was making big moves forward to accept my pain, I wasn't fully embracing 'acceptance'.

I still hadn't been totally honest with many of my friends, family and work colleagues about my chronic pain. When I look back, I am still surprised that I felt the need to hide it, but I think my attitude went back to the way society perceives chronic pain. I was afraid that people wouldn't believe me or accept my condition and I felt a sense of shame or weakness that I couldn't get rid of it; I felt like a failure that, despite all the treatment, medication and the biggest will in the world to be pain free, I wasn't. While I had resigned myself to living in pain, there was still a part of me that didn't fully accept the situation. Often my only outlet was my journal.

February 2010

Mask of pain

I am finding writing about my journey and experience with pain to be so upsetting, as I suppose every day I wear a mask that says, I am normal, life is good, I am getting on with day-to-day chores so I am OK ... but underneath that person everyone else sees is someone who is really struggling to do the simplest of tasks. I am finding getting in and out of the car a pain, typing at my desk in work a massive pain, going shopping, lifting my shopping into the car a pain and it depresses me. I ask why? WHY do I have pain? I ask myself this over and over again and I don't have the answer, so with all that internal struggle, the pain and the brain fog that living with chronic pain manifests, just living every day can be a very big problem. I feel my pain is slowly peeling off layers of my life, it can paralyse every aspect of my life and I have to ask myself, where is Andrea gone?

I am so sick and tired of crying tears for pain, I am angry with myself and my body. Why couldn't I stop this from happening? Honestly I don't really believe very many people care or even want to understand what someone with any type of chronic pain goes through daily. Occasions are marked by a pain score, I find myself remembering times past by how I was dealing with the pain.

I feel like there are two of us in this life: me and then pain, who is my secret twin who I seem to have to carry around with me all the time. Sometimes the load is easier: when I wake with a reduction in pain, I feel like a new person. With any reduction in pain I have a spring in my step, I get things done, I have sorted work issues, I actually find I'm wanting more out of every area of my life, particularly my personal relationship with my husband. I want to plan for date nights, holidays; without the pain I feel brave enough to travel in a car for a long journey to go somewhere, I want to have friends over, go out and be part of the hustle and bustle of the world. This is the life I want, this is the life I should have, this is the reason I feel so desperately robbed when the dreaded pain ramps up a gear and is in spasm or is back strongly, like it seems to be today in my coccyx area.

Why aren't people getting the support they need to deal with this problem? I think it is a fundamental human right to be able to live without daily pain. It is actually torture and it has to be stopped; people with pain are afraid to speak out, afraid to reveal their true feelings, afraid people will say it's 'all in your head'. I feel like saying to those people that it's all in my body, my life, my car, my bed, my shower, my work, my intimate relationships, my friendships. It is EVERYWHERE, so yes it does take a lot of space up in my brain because I can't do anything, even SLEEP, because it sneaks into my dreams: sometimes it's someone kicking me in the bum with a boot or sometimes I dream I have fallen and landed on my bum or even at times in my dreams I have been carrying a very heavy load that is almost making me fall, and when I wake from sleep PAIN is there in my shoulders, or my back or my bum.

SO as I sigh another sigh while writing this, trying to let the anger pass, I am back to where I have so much difficulty, the one thing I constantly struggle with that once again is back to haunt me – Andrea, just accept this is how it is, the elephant in the room, ACCEPTANCE.

This can be painful, not just physically, but emotionally. I struggle to accept this is my life. It is truly just too overwhelming to think about it always being with me. Today I am just exhausted with everything and the reality is tomorrow could be worse or, hopefully, better!

HOPE!

I suppose eventually the only way to deal with this effectively is to have some HOPE and also truly accept that, yes, the pain is there, but it's up to me, not a doctor, not a tablet or a miracle cure, to deal with it; it's me who has to start taking control of my life. I have this chat often with fellow chronic pain suffers about the feeling of hopelessness – sometimes we feel so deflated, dealing with the pain is just so consuming, but we can't allow pain to be our lives, it's just part of our lives. What is the old saying? Two things are certain in life, death and taxes – well for pain sufferers let's add a third, PAIN ... Stop fighting it, stop resenting and hating it, accept it as you would an old friend into your life. You probably know pain inside out if you've had it for a long time, or if you are at the beginning of your beautiful relationship with pain I have no doubt you know what makes it worse or eases it too. So rather than wasting energy wishing it away, or even trying to somehow control it – in my experience ultimately you can't control it, it comes without warning and can really flare up for no apparent reason – the lesson today is to just let it be and ACCEPT it. Once we have done that the challenge is what's next …

Sadly for me today, I think it's 1 to pain and 0 to me. I am so utterly wiped of energy, I just want to melt into this chair and somehow allow all my muscles to just turn into jelly. Even the thought of moving is too much of an effort today; I know that sounds over the top, but today is a great example of why I think pain sufferers allow themselves to be practically ignored by the government, medical professionals, even society: we just don't have the energy to fight. Sometimes I wish I had the energy to make a documentary on pain or even write a book to give some insight into a life in pain, but gathering the focus and drive to simply get out of the house on days when you aren't having a good pain day is a momentous task in itself.

I really would like to do an experiment to show people with no pain how it can affect your life, if only there was a scientific way to analyse the effect. I've always secretly wanted to get someone who is well known for their physical strength and endurance and, for one week, attach a zapping machine to various parts of their body to zap them with a little electric shock, randomly and sometimes persistently for a few hours or a few days and see what effect that has on their mood, concentration, motivation, on their basic ability to live day to day. It is almost impossible to truly know what it is like to live with pain unless you have experienced it on an ongoing basis. It truly breaks my heart to think of so many who have allowed the pain to win, who have isolated themselves, almost hidden themselves from society because no one believes them and they think they are the mad one – the loneliness and lack of empathy we have to endure is unacceptable. Shame on us as a society for not helping chronic pain sufferers more. Just as much as we as people with chronic pain have to accept we have it, society and the medical profession have to accept our pain is real and do something constructive to help us live with this and ensure we are treated as an equal part of society. For me now, my neck and head pain is almost unbearable so I have to accept that's all I can write for now. Andrea and her 'frenemy' pain are signing off.

10

A Different Person

When I look back to those early days and see where I am today, it seems like a world away. One thing is for sure – after I finished my pain management course I was a different person. By the end of the course, I was armed with brilliant tools that I could apply to my own life. I made lots of changes and I quickly saw the benefits.

Making the journey from the 'pain patient' to Andrea the person was a huge challenge at the start. But I had a secret goal that focused my mind – I wanted to start a family. I was determined, I was willing to put in the hard work, and in truth I was feeling very positive about the future. I think this was largely down to the support and understanding I now had around me that I had never had before. I knew it was okay to get angry, depressed and hopeless, that these feelings were normal. For the first time in my life when I felt that way I didn't bottle up those emotions and could reach out to people who understood me; the people on the pain management course had become my new 'pain friends'. We supported each other, even after the course finished – we will always share a special bond and many of us are still close friends to this day.

Another reason to feel hopeful about the future was the amazing 'care bubble' of medical specialists I now had to support me – my pain team of healthcare professionals that I had in place. I met with Dr Murphy after the pain management course and it was almost like my blinkers were off. Before the course I had wanted a complete absence of pain. However, now I realised the benefits of pain reduction and we talked about the value of pacing and following a daily pain plan. One of the biggest things he recognised was that I didn't have the right GP and he recommended Dr Penny Bleakley at the Beechlawn Medical Centre in Monkstown. He felt she would really help me manage my pain, and he was so right. Dr Bleakley has been amazing, she really understands chronic pain and is very caring and supportive. From our first meeting she listened attentively to me and my pain goals, she was very flexible and helpful with my approach to medication, and she still is to this day.

In our first appointment Penny got up to speed with my medical history (Dr Murphy had given her an overview of the procedures and medication I was on). She listened, she understood and she asked me what my goal was. I said I wanted to use everything I had learned to achieve the best possible life–pain–wellness balance. We talked about medication and I agreed to come back in a month's time and we could look at maybe reducing some medication then. I felt fantastic leaving the office. A doctor who understood and supported me – it was brilliant.

Penny had recommended a really good physiotherapist, Dr Marie Elaine Grant, who is an expert in managing chronic musculoskeletal pain. I started to go to physio weekly for core strengthening. Every week Dr Grant would push me just as much as I needed to be pushed. The weekly sessions boosted my confidence in what my body was capable of. I had had very low expectations of what I could do physically – which was partly fear and partly pain avoidance. I was afraid of the consequences of exercise on my pain. I felt this was a valid fear – in the past I had been to various people who didn't understand chronic pain and I had made my pain worse – but Dr Grant helped me with the weekly sessions and she suggested a brilliant Pilates teacher for me too. On her recommendation I made an appointment for a one-to-one session with Eva Berg, and to my surprise found she was based just down the road from me. Apart from being really knowledgeable, she is well tuned in to the realities of chronic pain. I began weekly Pilates classes and before long I was taking up to three classes a week. I felt stronger and I had a great sense of pride in myself for how far I had come.

I think the key to my success during that time was building my confidence, not only in myself, but also in the people guiding me. I felt confident that if anything was in any way dangerous to me or would cause additional pain, I had the experts in place to help me. I really put the work in to living a healthier life, and my daily walk and stretches, weekly Pilates and physio all became a regular part of my life. I also made time every day for relaxation through meditation, I tried to write regularly in my journal, I began to practise mindfulness and incorporated the cognitive behavioural therapy tools I learned to change my negative thought patterns and behaviours.

I made space and time each day for managing pain. Life became all about 'pacing and spacing' activities. Whereas in the past, if I had a low-pain day I might decide to clean the house from top to bottom or work late in the office, I could now see the patterns from my journal. I could see the benefits of pacing – doing things little and often rather than too much in one go. I could see that when I overdid things I would crash and burn, and be worse off for a week or two. For the first time I was starting to see the patterns, and this deeper understanding of chronic pain really helped me. When I felt a reduction in the daily pain, I could see what I might do to add to my wellness.

So with a few months of hard work, I had a new determination and a positive outlook on life. During this time I had wonderful support from my family and my 'pain friends' – they made the darker days a lot easier to handle – and a team of professionals who were willing me to do well and really helping me. I think they were genuinely invested in my wellness, too, and their support was invaluable.

Anyone with chronic pain will know that there are good days and bad. But now, when my pain flared up, instead of allowing my emotions to escalate to catastrophic thinking, I told myself, 'This will pass.'

Because I was really focused on wanting to start a family, I still had one big area to tackle – medication. I have always wanted to reduce my meds; ideally I would like to live without them completely. While medication has a very important role to play in the management of chronic pain, I have a very troubled relationship with my meds. I don't like some of their side effects and, if I could, I would choose not to take them at all, but that isn't always an option. At the time of writing this book I am on medication. If you are in a similar situation, any changes you want to make *must* be discussed with your healthcare professional.

When I met the other people on the pain management course I discovered that we were all on similar pain medication cocktails. We all knew each other's meds and we chatted about the effects, both positive and negative. It was very validating to know that other people had put on weight or felt they had brain fog from their meds, a loss of energy, loss of sex drive, dryness in the mouth, forgetfulness, memory difficulties or an inability to focus. We all agreed that the list of side effects seemed endless, and I realised it wasn't all in my imagination.

I had been on many different types of drug and I really wanted to reduce my intake. I made an appointment with my GP Penny to make a plan. I knew it was vital to be honest with her, and I felt that my pain journal gave a good picture of how I was coping.

I felt so positive when I went to see Penny. I had written a list of notes to share with her and I had a real hope that she would magically be able to make a big reduction in the tablets I was taking. In fact I felt so confident after my recent success with the pain management programme that I thought I could maybe even just stop taking some of them.

While there I mentioned that I was experiencing some pain in my thoracic area, which was a relatively new niggle. I also spoke very candidly about my desire to get pregnant. I wanted to work with her to reduce the medication slowly with the aim (hopefully) of being medication free in a few months, and then (hopefully) after that I would conceive.

Penny was a great support and gave me lots of hope. One of the wonderful things about Penny is her vast knowledge and understanding of both chronic pain and the pain management programme. She warned me that it might be tough, and stressed that I would have to put in the time and follow the programme: 'We want to avoid a flare-up, but if it happens we'll have to re-evaluate the medication and how it's working.'

The first thing to address was the spasm in the middle part of my back. She wanted to give me a muscle relaxant to try to settle that down, which was devastating news – I certainly wasn't expecting to be given extra medication. She was absolutely right, of course, as it could have really flared up if we didn't address it, but it wasn't part of my plan and the effect it had on me can be seen from my diary entry from the following day:

March 2010

I want my life back …
I had a very dark day yesterday, although I started the day well. I am working very hard on my pain management programme, and

I was feeling very good for all the changes that I have made in the last month.

As part of the pain management plan, I want to reduce my meds with the aim of completely coming off them altogether to try to get pregnant safely. This was my plan:

- *Seeing Dr Penny Bleakley*

- *New pain management plan*

- *Daily stretches*

- *Relaxation*

- *Walking*

- *Changing house around in process, moving things so no additional bending*

- *Appointments with Marie Elaine Grant (physio) & Eva Berg (Pilates) (already going really well, feeling stronger at my core)*

- *Also looking at changing my car*

Goals

- *Pain free*

- *Reduction of medication – my aim is to be off all by the end of the year*

- *Engaging and enjoying life more*

- *Starting a family*

- *Exploring alternative treatments for pain*

- *Document all med changes and also pain and lifestyle daily or weekly*

Pain-*free* Life

Issues

- *Sleep: still waking up every night in pain*
- *Very stiff/sore every morning, issues getting out of bed and starting the day*
- *Random spasms, mostly thoracic area*
- *Pain – various levels, definitely lower, though, in many areas*

Advice on

- *Reducing tablets*
- *Night-time sleep problems*
- *Low sex drive from tablets*

I was happily reading over my notes in the packed waiting room when my name was called.

'How have you been?' Penny asked.

'Really good,' I said. I explained that I was taking a break from my TV work so I was fully focused on my pain management programme and that I wanted to reduce my tablets. I explained that there was one I particularly hated – it made me feel not like myself, it made me fat, it killed my sex drive, it just made me feel 'off'. But on the positive side, it stopped the shooting nerve pain.

My right-side thoracic pain hadn't really eased, and it was waking me every night. Nights were probably the worst, as I would wake up feeling stiff and in pain. 'But these days I get out of bed. A few years ago I would have stayed in bed, but with my knowledge of chronic pain I force myself out of bed. A good cup of coffee from Dave usually kick starts my day and gets me out of bed. I know the pain will ease within an hour. A hot shower and movement helps.'

Penny listened to everything and said, 'We really need to sort out this muscle spasm', so before long she was advising me to take another tablet in the short term.

I said, 'I want to stop taking tablets. I wanted a big drop-down, but I only managed to get a small reduction, and now I have to take an extra one, when I just want to stop taking any?'

'Why do you want to stop taking your medication?' Penny asked.

'I want to start a family, because I want to feel like me again!' Suddenly I was in tears. I blurted out that when I was in the waiting room there were two new mums holding tiny babies and I was thinking that if I had a baby I probably wouldn't even be able to hold it properly, because of this pain. 'Penny, I'm sorry for getting upset. It's just so hard, it's very difficult to stay positive. I'm really working hard and my goal from today was to come off the tablets. I need to feel like I have some control over my life.'

Penny was, and always is, so understanding. We took a moment to go through my current medication and we looked at a time frame of a couple of months to reduce the medication I was currently on. I agreed to make an appointment for one month later and I dried my tears, regained my composure and said my goodbyes.

After the consultation I walked to my car, looked at the long list of drugs I needed to get and I felt a veil of sadness come over me. My happy mood was gone. As I studied the list of tablets I realised that in addition to what I was taking already, there was a new one for spasms.

No matter how super positive I had been on the way to the doctor, and despite all the work that I had been doing on my pain management programme, I still wasn't in control. I went in with the goal of reducing my medication, so it was just soul-destroying to come out with more tablets to take. Then, just thinking about the next few days, how truly terrible my body would feel as I introduced a new tablet and the adverse effects of withdrawal as I reduced one of my other tablets, made me feel utterly hopeless. Sometimes, even weeks after introducing a new tablet you can feel rotten. Will they suit my system? Will I have side effects? Will I get more tablet fog?

I sat in the car and looked down at the prescription, a reminder that something is wrong in my body. Hard as I try, I can't seem to help or heal myself. I don't have control. I have to take these tablets, then there's the pain too – the tablets don't even get rid of all the pain. I just feel that every little thing I do, every bloody part of my life, is taken over by pain: taking tablets, feeling sore, feeling out of control. It's crap, it's lonely and it's sad. The tears flowed again and I thought, 'I'm sitting here in my car enveloped by sadness. I don't feel I can drive, I can't call anyone to talk about my feelings. All I can do is sit as this sinks in. I have reduced the tablets slightly but I also have another chemical to add to the toxic cocktail of medication I have to endure.'

As I sat in silence, time seemed to disappear. I don't know how long I was sitting there. I sat in a trance, watching the fast-moving traffic motoring past. I noticed in my mirror that one car was driving particularly fast and for a split second – I feel so ashamed to even write this – I thought about just stepping out and getting hit by a car. I had never considered anything like that before. I was thinking at that moment that, if I did that, I would go to hospital and my pain would be visible in my injuries. In that moment of madness, I felt that there was no end, no solution to the pain, it had taken my work, my intimate relationship, my positive outlook on life, it had taken me. Andrea had gone, lost behind this medication. My mood was so dark I was even losing my will to live, although I knew intellectually I had so much to live for.

Amazingly, just as I looked out of my car window at the speeding car zooming by, a church bell rang out! I found a pen and wrote this on the back of my receipt from the doctor:

I feel safer now, I know I am not alone, God is always here.

I call upon my guardian angel, St Bridget, Archangel Michael and Raphael and Gabriel and any angels who want to help me today. I need to lift my vibration, I need to feel positive again, I need to feel safe and secure, I know I am blessed, loved and protected by heaven and the universe.

I feel my dad is here too. I love you, Dad, allow me to feel your loving presence, please show me a sign from heaven this day. I know you and all the angels and saints are with me, guiding me safely on my divine path in life. Helping me along, revealing why I have this constant pain. I will wait and watch.

It sounds so ridiculous, but a ray of sunshine filled the sky with a beautiful bright glow and I did feel happier. I could see the steeple in the distance, so I decided to drive up to the church. I wasn't even sure if it would be open. There were no parking spots, so I decided to make a U-turn to look again, and, as luck would have it, there was a parking space, perfectly positioned in front of the church. I was still in tears as I parked and walked into the beautiful empty church. I had never been in it before; it was in the village of Monkstown in Dublin. I knelt at a statue of Padre Pio and prayed. This was the saint Dad had prayed to and I associate his prayers and blessings with my father.

As I prayed in silence, I noticed there was a book for special petitions.

So I wrote, as the tears flowed uncontrollably, that I wanted to pray for all the people in this world experiencing pain. I asked heaven to bless them and have mercy on them, brighten their road ahead so they could see that life isn't all about pain. I waited in the church for about half an hour, praying and looking around for something – some sign to fill me with hope.

Eventually I made my way to the door, happier after praying and lighting lamps, and hoping that my prayer to conceive would be answered. As I walked to the car, I suddenly had a moment of clarity. Something suddenly made sense. I thought, 'Maybe I can't control the pain, but I can control my thoughts, and your thoughts create your future! So I'm going to visualise myself well and pain free and pregnant, feeling healthy and full of joy. This new tablet is a minor issue, it will help the spasm and I will be off it and I will reduce the other tablets.'

11

Prayers Answered

So there wasn't to be a quick fix. Any reduction in my meds would happen over a number of months.

My dream to get pregnant hadn't started as I'd hoped. I was temporarily on a new tablet, but I was confident that this was just a minor setback. Eventually I did come off that tablet, reducing the dosage gradually, month by month. And, with Penny's help, after a number of months I was off all my medication. Hurrah!

I continued regular Pilates with Eva Berg, who was a great confidante. I told her of my plans and she really helped me work on my core. She also advised me which moves on the reformer machine wouldn't be advisable for my back, and she gave me stretches to do at home.

Physiotherapist Dr Marie Elaine Grant continued to see me, and we made really good progress each week, using a variety of treatments to help me deal with increased pain from the reduction in medication. Each week I also had a number of routine stretches to do at home, which helped strengthen my core. I also tried a number of alternative treatments to help alleviate my pain: a TENS machine, massage, reflexology, energy healing, Reiki, cupping, tapping. You name it, I tried it! I can't say that many of these are still part of my daily pain management plan, but at the time they probably helped me a little.

Workwise, I made a conscious effort to take it easy. Luckily enough I was on a freelance contract with TV3 for *Animal A&E*,

so, unlike many other presenters who are staff, I didn't have to be in the building every day. Until we started shooting the next series I had the summer months off and I didn't pursue any new work. On a week to week basis I had my voice-over continuity work, which required a few hours two days a week, and my Saturday show with Sunshine 106.8, but for the rest of the week I really focused on my wellness and my desire to achieve my dream of becoming pregnant.

I tried to stay as positive as possible and I made a conscious effort every day to find the joy in life again. I would seek out things that brought me joy. I spent a lot of time walking and observing nature, and I prayed constantly. I prayed for a miracle, I prayed for strength, I prayed for healing, I prayed for heaven's assistance. During my daily walk I would repeat my positive affirmations – I would be pain free, I would be off tablets and I would have a healthy baby.

In the past, when people asked us about starting a family, I would brush the comment off, pretend it wasn't for me at the moment, and many times this was actually true, as I knew that getting pregnant wasn't safe while I was taking daily medication and often getting injections under X-ray. Sometimes, I felt hopeless and helpless inside and totally depressed about my situation.

But now something had switched in me. When someone asked me during those few months, I would say, 'Yes, I'm going to get pregnant very soon.' I would even go as far as saying how excited I was and I would almost allow my body to feel the joy I would experience if I were pregnant. I know a few people felt I was a little crazy, but that's how I felt.

Honestly? I was in pain, I can't say I wasn't. But I was pacing and I was really working the pain management programme, and I had had a mental shift – the fear of pain was gone. It no longer controlled me. I was in charge at last.

I spoke to my husband about my scientific plan for getting pregnant. At this time I had been off all the medication for maybe a month or two and my pain was manageable but increasing, so I decided next month would be when I wanted to concentrate on conceiving. I truly believed it was going to happen and I had researched the best method to get pregnant successfully. I purchased an ovulation predictor kit and we had a busy month, at the end of which, on Sunday 31 October 2010, to our huge surprise we discovered we were pregnant. That day David and I walked with Dash in a beautiful park in Dublin. The autumn sun was shining as we strolled almost in a trance; I don't think we could believe it, so we didn't really talk too much about it. We just walked hand in hand in silence. I was thrilled, shocked, nervous, surprised and worried. I prayed in thanksgiving – 'Thank you for this miracle' – and, most of all, I prayed that this miracle would stay alive in my body.

We decided I should book to see my GP Penny, followed by my physio, and then I would see my Pilates teacher. I saw Penny the next day, we did the test and she said, 'Congratulations! Yes you are!' and we both beamed at each other. Then I blurted out to Penny that I was really worried because of the pain. With the pregnancy, I wouldn't be able to take medication. Then I thought of all the medication I had taken in the past – that might affect the baby. I was worried about everything!

Penny said the most amazing and beautiful thing, and I shall never forget it (thinking of her words now still fills me with happiness). 'You're a mum now, trust me, you're always going to be worried. It's normal for anybody who's expecting to be worried: worried about pregnancy, the delivery, bringing baby home, crawling, walking … That's what parents do – they worry!'

We smiled and I cried. She said, 'We'll manage the pain', and we spoke about hospitals. She recommended a great doctor in Holles Street.

And that was that. I was having a baby! My prayers had been answered – thank you, God.

So this was when the serious pain management kicked in for me. Once again I tried to stay positive and focused on the beautiful miracle growing inside me. I didn't want to tell anybody for as long as possible as I feared that something might go wrong.

I had a day of panic midway through my pregnancy, when a journalist sent me a message on Facebook saying, 'Congratulations on your new arrival!' I was rarely in the papers unless it was about a case of animal neglect from the TV show and I certainly didn't want this to end up in the gossip section of a Sunday newspaper. Most of all, I really didn't want anyone to know until I was ready to share the news. Fortunately, my dear friend Valerie Roe, who works in PR, explained to the journalist – whom she knew – about our situation, my concerns about my chronic pain and my desire not to share the news, and asked that they pull the story. It wasn't printed, which was a huge relief. Each day and month that passed, I felt relief, and each milestone – the twelve-week and twenty-week scans – made me feel a bit safer in the knowledge that my baby was thriving.

Pain wise, I didn't complain once while I was pregnant. I felt so blessed to be pregnant that I just accepted more pain as I grew bigger. During my pregnancy I really perfected my practice of relaxation and breathing, and I used this daily to help with the pain.

At work I had begun to shoot the new series of *Animal A&E*. It was a particularly cold winter, we were travelling the country and it was a very challenging time for me. I really wanted to get to the end of the series shoots before mentioning it to anyone. I planned to tell my colleagues when I had finished the last day of shooting. I managed to schedule only one rescue a week so in between filming I was resting. We had an amazing crew on that series. I was given great flexibility and support; in fact it was practically an all-female team, a great camerawoman Joan, Cat our brilliant director and the ever helpful Graham on sound.

What proved to be our last day of shooting was very upsetting and challenging. We were in Lower Killeens in Cork and the weather had been very cold with heavy snow and frost – unusual for the beginning of March. I was with Lisa O'Donovan from the ISPCA on an abandoned horse investigation. The field where we wanted to film ran along the bank of a river. We were investigating a claim that two horses had been abandoned and after the recent cold snap would be left to suffer and possibly die without urgent intervention. It was a difficult place to navigate as it was marshy land with heavy gorse bushes. We searched for the horses, believing that they might have gone into the gorse for shelter. It was a dangerous rescue and, not only was I pregnant, I also had a lot of pain that day. I had to be careful and I had great support from a wonderful crew. But, like Lisa, my mind was focused on the poor horses.

We walked for a distance through the overgrown gorse bushes when the vet who was assisting us noticed what he believed to be an aborted foetus. One of the horses had been in foal. It was so shocking and upsetting and it had a huge effect on me. I decided then that this would have to be my last rescue and my last day working on location while I was pregnant. Luckily the story had a happy ending: the two horses were located in the scrub and we managed to save them both. On returning to TV3, I told my producer I wouldn't be able to go on any more rescues because I was over five months pregnant.

From the six-month mark onwards I continued with some

voice-over work and my Saturday radio show, but I rested a lot. Every time my pain increased I would remind myself of the miracle growing inside. That's when I realised that pain is an emotion, but so is love. The love for my unborn child was stronger than my feelings of pain.

I had also been working on an ongoing basis since we started the animal show on two documentaries that I was passionate about, but we hadn't any guarantee that they would be given the green light. Following my work over the years on *Animal A&E*, I wanted to highlight both the issue of puppy farming and the abandoned horse crisis in Ireland that had unfolded in recent years. The plan for these stand-alone documentaries would be to air them at prime time, but later than *Animal A&E*: these hour-long programmes would be more hard-hitting. We had been working away on them for months and I was really determined to get them to air, hoping that highlighting the issues might help change the puppy farming and equine laws in this country.

I felt we needed to highlight the cruelty I had witnessed while we were filming, so I was thrilled when we did get a transmission date and the go-ahead to complete them, but, typical of TV schedules, the delivery date was brought forward and my two delivery dates were clashing! I found myself finishing the documentaries when I was thirty-eight weeks pregnant. Luckily this only involved recording the in-vision links to camera, since a lot of the footage had already been shot during the previous series. I had a great team of people, who made the work easy, plus great support from my husband and family, but it was tough and rewarding in equal measure. I knew that within weeks my own little miracle would soon be in the world too.

June 2011 Gratitude Diary

Thank you, God, Angels and Universe for my wonderful husband, Dash, my family, my friends. I am feeling so thankful and excited about the new life that is about to enter the world. I have finished work today, I am on maternity leave! I am so grateful and overjoyed to be finished as I know we will meet our daughter soon. I am feeling truly blessed. Continue to watch over us. Thank you. A x

12

New Life is Born

I felt so blessed to be pregnant that I prayed every day to have a good birth and deliver a healthy child. Despite the later complications, both my prayers were answered.

My lower-back pain made it difficult to distinguish my normal pain from pregnancy-related pain. I went over my due date by a day or two, but the time finally arrived when I felt it was the right time to go to the hospital. I had felt an unusual sensation of pressure and, being a first-time mum, I was nervous and unsure. So we headed into the hospital, excited about the prospect of our new arrival.

At the hospital I definitely felt a contraction and I was a little nauseous, but I had my trusted methods of dealing with pain. I was doing my visualisation, breathing, exercises and relaxation, and I even had a shower – water can be very relaxing and soothing. Almost in a meditative state, I walked slowly up the corridor to the room where I would give birth and asked if I could go to the toilet. The nurse waited outside. I was having a contraction and I felt I needed to relax my mind and breathe through the pain. Because I was taking a while, the nurse became worried, so she asked me when I had had my last contraction. I said that actually I had just had it. She didn't know whether to believe me because I was being so calm and quiet!

Things became more intense after that and within thirty minutes I had an anaesthetist on hand to give me an epidural. For people with chronic back pain, needles go hand in hand with pain relief, so when he sat me forward and began the procedure I didn't move, but immediately I felt a sharp pain at the base of my skull and I suddenly became very vocal, I knew something had happened but wasn't sure what. Then I felt a pain in the top of my leg, at that point I knew the needle had gone in wrong – and probably gone in wrong twice. After a number of attempts the epidural eventually went in, but I could feel intense pain immediately. Unless this has happened to you, you can't understand the pain. It was unbearable. I felt as though my head was crashing down on my neck.

What had happened was unfortunate. It can happen occasionally, but it is rare. It seems that the thin membrane that surrounds the spinal cord was punctured by the epidural needle; when this happens there is a possibility of leaking spinal fluid. The fluid acts as a cushion around the brain and without it, the brain tends to sag and rubs against the skull, which causes severe pain – it's called an epidural headache. So before I even pushed, I had this awful pain.

Mercifully, it was a very short labour and, within an hour, our Brooke was born. It was 6.05 p.m. on 12 July 2011. It had all happened so fast, and it was the happiest and proudest day of my life. My doctor and the midwife were both amazing, it was very calm and almost everything about the delivery worked out perfectly.

But just after she was born, I had to address the pain in my head. It was severe, an eight on the pain scale, whereas the contractions had been maybe seven or eight. And it was getting worse; sitting up made it worse and lights seemed to affect it too.

For some reason I was brought right back to when I was a fifteen-year-old in Cherry Orchard Hospital, the night when I had a headache and pain after the lumbar puncture, when I knew something had gone wrong but didn't know what it was. The next day I had had a very bad headache and pain in my lower back and I clearly remember a nurse saying it was period pains.

Back to the present, and I knew that something was seriously wrong. I became very vocal and told the staff that things weren't right, that I needed something for serious pain. I was in so much pain that David had to give Brooke her first feed, her first bath, change her first nappy. The first night was awful. David was exhausted, both physically and emotionally, so he went home to sleep. He left very late, around 11 p.m.

I had been due to get tablets from the nurses but there was some mix-up and it wasn't written in my chart that I should have pain relief. I ended up texting my sister Lavinia in the UK to ask my brother-in-law, the doctor, what I should do for the pain. By 3 a.m. I was in tears, alone with my beautiful baby beside me. The pain was excruciating. It was at the base of my neck and it felt really serious. I had some Nurofen that David had brought to the hospital for himself and I took them. The text back from Lavinia advised me to drink Coke if I had it – and there was some in David's little bag of goodies he had bought in the shop. Apparently the caffeine in Coke will often temporarily relieve the pain associated with this type of headache because it increases the production of cerebrospinal fluid (CSF) in the brain.

The lowest point came that night when Brooke needed to be picked up. This tiny, delicate, perfect little angel needed her mother. I sat up and managed to pick her up in my arms and rest her on my chest. It was so painful I cried.

It was a really difficult first night. When the nurse came into me in the morning I had a pillow over my head – the light in the shared room was flashing and made the headache worse – and Brooke lying beside me. It had been the longest night of my life, one I wouldn't want to repeat. It had robbed me of the enjoyment of nurturing my first-born daughter. Once again pain had taken centre stage in my life. The anger, along with the pain and hormones, took quite a toll.

Things improved quickly when my doctor arrived early that morning. Immediately a pain control plan was put in place and I was given the care and attention I needed. Brooke's proud daddy and both her nans were standing by to dote on her and make sure she had all the love and care she needed.

Things were surely looking up. She was an angel, as quiet as a mouse and so good, I felt she was heaven-sent. Although I couldn't really pick her up – I had to stay flat on my back – I had a wonderful and precious gift, a healthy baby. I kept my spirits high by constantly reminding myself that lying beside me was the answer to my prayers.

My first immediate challenge after the birth was getting the correct treatment for the post-epidural headache. I can't really call it just a headache; this was more severe, unlike any headache I had ever experienced. I had lots of discomfort, pain and pressure, not only at the base of my head, but down into my neck and shoulder area as well. I felt queasy and the bright hospital lights made me feel worse. The first treatment advised was to simply lie flat on my back, and this seemed to ease the pain slightly, but as soon as I stood up it was a lot worse. This, apparently, is due to a persistent leak of spinal fluid into the epidural space.

I was also told to drink plenty of fluid. Surprisingly, drinks containing caffeine, such as tea, coffee and cola, are especially helpful. Caffeine is not a cure but it does give some relief. Caffeine is a vasoconstrictor, which means that it makes blood vessels contract. Reducing the flow of blood into the brain means that there is a consequent easing of pressure on the cerebrospinal fluid. It seemed strange to be knocking back can after can of Red Bull and drinking coffee, particularly as I hadn't had coffee all through the pregnancy, so all the caffeine made me feel totally out of sorts. And despite an extra day in hospital lying flat on my back, there was no change in my pain levels.

More than anything, I wanted to hold my beautiful new daughter. Like most expectant mothers, I had spent ages imagining how it would be after giving birth. I imagined precious time bonding with my daughter, lots of cooing, oohing, aahing, and night feeds – like Eavan Boland's poem. I hadn't factored in additional pain and being forced to lie flat. Dealing with the pain was difficult enough, and it's an emotional time anyway – as most mothers can understand – but being unable to nurse Brooke was the hardest thing for me to handle.

The pain management team at Holles Street Hospital advised that I should get an epidural blood patch – the best treatment for a post-dural puncture headache. It isn't for the faint-hearted and I must admit I wasn't looking forward to it. It is carried out while you are fully awake. A large blood sample is taken from your arm, then your own blood is injected into your back, near the hole in the dura, and straight into the epidural space that has been punctured. The aim is to 'plug the leak' and then the headache should go away.

All through the first procedure I prayed to Archangel Gabriel. For some reason, since Brooke's birth I felt the urge to direct my prayers to him. All I could think of was holding Brooke. I was desperate to bring her home, to cradle and hold her, and begin our family life – this is what kept me focused throughout the procedure, which took about half an hour. In the end it wasn't too uncomfortable; you just feel a pressure building in your spine at the location where the blood is injected.

Soon after my first blood patch I returned home and hoped the headache would ease. I had been told that most patients experience significant relief immediately. Unfortunately, for me that wasn't the case. Despite more rest and lying flat on my back at home, the headache persisted and I had to return to the hospital for another blood patch procedure. Again it wasn't fully successful. I was feeling very discouraged and still in pain. It was very hard on David, too, as he had to do the daily grind of nappy changing and round-the-clock feeds, as well as taking me back and forth to the hospital, so sleep deprivation was a massive strain on him during those first few days.

Finally a decision was made to take me to St Vincent's Hospital and repeat the procedure under X-ray, using a fluid to see exactly where the puncture was. It was a success of sorts – the headache was rectified, but I was left with a lot of neck pain and pain at the base of my head. Nevertheless, I felt so happy. I was a mum and we were a family! My family life was just perfect and so was my daughter, Brooke Rose Torpey.

August 2011

Despite the pain today I have to make a really conscious effort to be happy and grateful. I feel blessed for so many positives in my life, every day I say thank you for my wonderful family. Just looking at Baby Brooke fills me with joy.

One of the things that I find hard about having chronic pain and being a mother and wife is the effect it has on those around me that I love. I feel sad for David, I know it's not easy for him to watch me in pain. I know certain things need to be considered before we travel or make plans, or just doing a very normal thing like carrying my beautiful daughter can cause extra pain. I find I am asking myself do I carry her as much as other mothers do with their children? With the pain in my neck and shoulders still lingering I am thinking about going back on my tablets again, but even as I write this I am also very aware of the effect taking tablets has had on me in the past and the knock-on effects it has had on my relationship with David. I know he has seen clearly how tablets affect my mood, my energy, my libido, my life, his life – our life! So if I think about this I can get very down.

A new and very upsetting development is the thought of my daughter seeing me in pain, particularly if I am unable to pick her up when she gets bigger. Will she be aware of mummy being sick? Should I hide it from her? As she gets older I know she will pick up on it. Lately I have been thinking about how I can explain the pain to her. She will be too young to properly understand it for a few years, but it will be a conversation I will have to have.

More recently I have worried that maybe she might experience pain. This is a terrible fear. I know there is no proof to show that this pain is hereditary but what if it is?

I am hoping that writing about these fear-based thoughts will help me to have clarity that they are irrational. In truth, until I had Brooke I hadn't given much thought to how pain might affect my parenting! I have to make a real effort to choose happy thoughts every day and remind myself just how lucky I am. xxx

13

Being Mum

At last I could start to settle into motherhood and caring for my precious new baby, Brooke. We battled the usual struggles of first-time parents. Sleep was a distant memory, which I found okay as I wasn't used to restful sleep anyway, but physically and emotionally we were both drained. As a couple we quickly discovered that, no matter how carefully we had discussed and planned for parenthood, there were things we still needed to work through and simply couldn't predict or plan for. Brooke had reflux, which presented some extra challenges.

Despite the lack of sleep, the added pressure and responsibility of caring for this helpless new person and, of course, my own personal physical recovery from giving birth, I can honestly say it was the most joyous time in our lives. We all bonded and David and I loved getting to know our new daughter. In those first few weeks we got lots of great support from Brooke's nans, who were both on hand to help.

In no time I settled into life as a mother and I loved it. I woke up one morning with the overwhelming feeling that my sole purpose in this life was to give birth to Brooke, to bring her into the world. I suddenly thought, 'Am I here so Brooke could be born?' I felt that her mission on earth would be formidable, so maybe my biggest mission was to be a good mother. I prayed in thanksgiving to God, I gave thanks for the blessing of my daughter. If my life purpose was to be a good, supportive, caring, nurturing mother, or maybe even a mother with flaws so that Brooke could learn crucial lessons for her purpose in life, then that's what would happen. An overwhelming understanding of unconditional love washed over me. I felt truly blessed. I was so happy and content.

For the most part I wanted to forget about my pain, to push it to the back of my mind and focus on Brooke and on being a mum. In truth it's just not that easy. Even when you ignore pain, it doesn't give up. Every day my brain was processing pain, and with constant pain you have other challenges too. Slowly but surely it drains all your energy. There is no recovery time and it isn't just one day of severe pain – it's permanent. My plan to ignore it just wasn't going to work.

Since giving birth my back pain had been quite severe, and I still had neck and head pain. I found it hard to carry out even the simplest daily activities, particularly carrying the car seat and getting Brooke in and out of it. One moment really stands out for me. I was bringing Brooke to the local public health nurse for her three-month developmental review. I arrived for the appointment a little flustered as we were running slightly late. Normally, I would carry her into the clinic in the car seat with a blanket over her, but I physically couldn't get the car seat out of the car. I just didn't have the upper body strength. I was in such a rush I just carried her in my arms and wrapped the blanket around her.

When we finally got to see the lovely nurse I tried to explain what had happened and found myself telling her how hard I was finding things. I hadn't quite considered how difficult it was going to be to manage my chronic pain routine, which I had been following religiously, and deal with the challenges that come with being a mum and Brooke's ever-changing routine of feeding and sleeping. I confided to the nurse that I found picking up Brooke very difficult and that, because the baby routine was so demanding and unpredictable, I had let my own daily pain routine go out the window. I am not sure she fully grasped the concept of chronic pain – perhaps she thought it was just the general aches and pains that go hand in hand with being a new mum – but I knew from my emotional outburst that I wasn't managing well. I needed to get on top of the pain.

After a few days I finally decided to book an appointment to see my GP, Penny. I was desperately trying to pretend that the pain wasn't an issue. I didn't want to deal with it – I almost felt I couldn't complain about the pain because Brooke was here and, after all, my prayers had been answered. But the pain seemed to be getting worse.

November 2011

Take action!

Stop sitting on the fence! Take action today!

It doesn't matter what you do as long as you do something. Energy is movement, and once you are in motion your positive thoughts & angels can focus energy towards your heart's desires.

So today I pick my angel card and it is to 'take action'.

I had a manic morning, although even before the day began it was already a bad start. Yesterday afternoon I could feel the pain increasing. I always have pain, but I did notice the intensity building up, which isn't good. By the end of the day, I couldn't even text on my mobile as I was in excruciating pain. It was very bad, I woke up a few times during the night in pain. I had strange dreams too. I was dreaming I was washing my hands and my fingers were sore and cut. I can't really remember it all, but my day was off to a bad start, the pain was moving from my head into my arms and hands and it was clearly affecting me, even when sleeping.

Pain-*free* Life

I got up, started the morning routine of feeding, washing, dressing Brooke, and got the baby bag ready for Mary's. While Brooke was playing happily, I got myself ready. I was putting on my clothes, which seemed to take for ever, even trying to get my socks on was a massive chore. Feeling under pressure time-wise, I was stressed, trying to carry things downstairs and I dropped my coffee. This is happening a lot to me, so to add to everything I had a little cleaning added to my morning routine. I didn't even manage make-up this morning. I notice when my neck, head and arms are sore I often drop things: it feels like my grip is weaker.

Anyway we eventually got out the door. I had Dash with me too as I was going to bring him for his walk in the park after dropping Brooke in to see Nanny Mary, who said she would be happy to mind her for a few hours so I could get a few things done. I got Brooke into the car seat and into the car with the baby bag, got the lead for Dash, put him in the boot, went back to get my bag and closed the front door. I suddenly realised I didn't have car keys, which also had my house keys with them, so we were locked out. I tried around the back but that door was locked too. Luckily our neighbours had a spare set, so eventually we got into the car to start our day, but I was drained. I am convinced pain stops certain parts of your brain from functioning properly, or else it is baby brain! I was a little late dropping Brooke – it just takes so long for me to get up and ready and out the door. This is normal for all first-time mums, lots of my friends share similar stories, but I just feel with the pain I wake up exhausted. I feel like I have drunk a bottle of wine. Thank God I am not drinking at the moment.

In truth, though, whatever pain plan I have isn't working, I am not sleeping and only for Brooke I would probably be in bed. It's hard to know if this is just the norm for a new parent. All day my mind has been going over this. I managed to drag myself around the park. Dash didn't get into the dog park today as I really didn't feel like talking to other people. As I walked around the park, though, I noticed that my head was really sore and sensitive. I had earphones on and the head bit of the earphones was actually really sore against my head. This shouldn't happen, because it's a very light touch and really the pain I am feeling is not matching up to the action causing the pain. This is a classic thing with chronic pain; sometimes people who don't suffer from chronic pain can't and will never understand. If I was with someone today and said to them, my head is really sore from the headphones, they would think I was crazy, but it was actually very sore. I only realised it was the headphones when I started moving them around and noticed that when the pressure was less or displaced to a different part of my head it eased a little. That actually is crazy. So often when you have chronic pain, your pain senses are heightened so that something that shouldn't hurt you really does. If you constantly complain people will think you are mad, because it doesn't make sense – how could earphones hurt? I will say they don't always hurt, but today my neck, arms and head are very achy, it kind of makes me feel like vomiting. Again that sounds very over the top, but that's honestly how I feel. I am really aware writing this that I rarely, if ever, write down how I am actually feeling in great detail, and I rarely really tell anyone, I just get on with life and accept it. Today my head feels fuzzy, heavy, delicate, truly the only thing it reminds me of is being hung-over, a pain hangover! Lovely, just what I needed.

As I walk around the park my mind turns back to Brooke, she is my life's purpose now. Since having my daughter I really notice I do get out of bed easier, she is my reason to fight this pain every day and try to live the best that I can. So what 'action' am I going to take? I am going to call Penny in the morning and book an appointment to talk about how I am coping, or not coping, as the case may be. Quite simply, my pain level is really up today, and it makes everything so hard. I need to be honest and ask for help.

As I sat in the waiting room I was going over in my head what I might say to Penny. I was thinking about Brooke, my gorgeous little daughter who was growing and getting heavier each week; she was on the move, too, so maybe I was just wearing myself out. I needed to talk to Penny about the increased pain in my head, neck and thoracic area. I wasn't sure if this was from what happened with the epidural or if it was the additional pressure on my body from lifting car seats, baby bags and generally being a mum. Maybe it was a mixture of both. My name was called and I found myself in a familiar place, sitting in front of Penny. And, yes, I was crying. She only had to ask 'How are you?' to set me off.

Of course I knew where I was going wrong. I hadn't been following any pain management plan; in truth, I had no plan, no systems in place. Now I had more pain than ever before and pain in new areas. My upper back was probably worse than my lower back now. I was feeling desperate. I knew only too well that the pain cycle of flare-up after flare-up had begun again and I wasn't sleeping or enjoying life much. But at the same time I felt like a fraud saying all this to Penny, because I was truly over the moon about being a mum. I was just finding it hard to cope.

So we had a chat and decided that we needed to get the pain under control and to address the lack of sleep. Brooke was starting to sleep more through the night but I wasn't sleeping at all much because of my increased pain. So I was given some of the old familiar medications, and there was also a new one. I got the prescription and started the tablets. You generally start low and quickly build up. At the start it's all good, as it takes a while to experience any adverse effects, and I suppose I was hoping this would be the magic combination of tablets that wouldn't need altering and wouldn't have any side effects. Of course, that was wishful thinking, but it helped in the meantime and got me back on track.

14

Trying to Juggle it All

For the next year life was so busy with my daughter and work that I just kept taking the tablets, trying to deal with the pain and trying to keep going. I was in unfamiliar territory. I was back at work, busy filming *Animal A&E*; and whereas before I would push myself hard on a shoot, safe in the knowledge that I could come home and take a few days to recover, there was no recovery time now. I was a busy mum with an active toddler, so it was all go, go, go.

I loved my role as a parent and for me that came before my pain. However, the reality of dealing with chronic pain soon overtakes even the most positive and determined person. I knew the burden of pain was wearing me down and I realised if I didn't look after myself I wouldn't be much good to Brooke. As Albert Einstein said, the definition of insanity is doing the same thing over and over again and expecting different results. I knew that to feel better and manage better I needed to make big changes.

I think I soon realised that the tablets were not enough, so I decided to go back to Dr Murphy to try to tackle the neck and arm pain. We started the familiar blocks, rhizotomies and pulsed radio frequency (PRF) treatments and I hoped that we could crack the pain. However, deep down I knew why I wasn't getting a whole lot better. I was – kind of – managing, bumping along, but I knew I would be in a bad place sooner rather than later if I didn't address the pain and how I was dealing with it.

After a number of months I suggested to Dr Murphy that I would like to do the pain management course again. It was over two years since I had last been on it, but I really felt it would help me. I had such a positive experience the first time and ultimately it was the catalyst for me being strong enough to go off my medication to conceive Brooke, so I felt confident that it was exactly what I needed. My life was so different now. I had different demands and pressures, and I had increased pain in my upper neck, shoulders and arms. So I asked Dr Murphy to put me forward for the course.

As before, I needed to be assessed for my suitability. In addition to the hospital approval I needed a letter from Penny to say I was fit enough to take part. She thought it was a great idea and felt it would be good for me too. Once again I was put through my paces by the hospital physiotherapist. This time there were some new assessments: I had to walk lengths at a fast speed for ten minutes, roll on a bed, step up and down on steps, move from sitting to standing – lots of different challenges to test my level of fitness. Unlike the first time round, I really applied myself and didn't complain too much.

Next stop was the occupational therapist, who felt like a trusted friend at this stage. I had stayed in touch with Blonny Brennan after the first course so it was so lovely to see her again and catch up. I was relieved when she said that I was very wise to want to come back. She agreed that my life had changed after having my daughter so, naturally, there would be lifestyle adjustments needed and, as my priorities had changed, I would benefit from doing the course a second time.

Finally I met clinical psychologist, Rosemary Walsh. Again I felt very at ease chatting to her. I never really know if there is an agenda at this stage, as it feels as though you are just chatting.

Thankfully, I was deemed suitable to do the course, and I found myself once again based in the hospital for three weeks. While the course was pretty much the same, it felt different because I had different goals and different reasons for being there. But, however diverse the group of pain sufferers, you know you all share a common bond that ties you together. In that group you will find compassion, support, understanding and a shoulder to cry on or someone to laugh along with. And, most importantly, no judgement.

November 2012

I have been checked in, I am wearing my designer hospital gown and have my net pants on and I am waiting. I am also praying, but today I just feel angry.

How many times have I prayed, have I tried to make a pact with God saying please make this go away?

I will do anything, God, please take it away!

When I am in flare-up I find nothing makes sense, I feel over-whelmed, not in control. I need to get control of other areas of my life because this is so unpredictable. At least I can recognise the signs now and try to avoid the panic that sets in.

I always second guess myself. I'm somebody who believes so strongly in being positive, I read endless books that say you can achieve anything you want if you believe it and work hard, focus, keep your goal in mind! So what am I doing wrong? I've written in diaries that I'm healthy, pain free, happy and fit. I've tried not to talk about it, I've desperately tried to pretend all my positive thinking will heal me, but sadly it's never gone away ... yet!

I'm sitting here in the day ward of St Vincent's, barely able to write, listening to the sound of the rain, and I am desperately trying to find a reason why I have this chronic never-ending elusive pain. I believe everything happens for a reason but it's so hard to understand any reason for my pain. Please someone help me, please someone help me, please someone help me, I don't want to feel like this. Pain makes me feel very old, I feel like my body is letting me down, or am I letting my body down?

Could I do something to change this cycle of pain? I need answers. I put a brave face on, but I feel today I can't take any more. I don't know what more to do!

Pain management courses, ongoing injections, healers, meditating, what works? I am feeling deflated in a way that I am starting my second pain management course on Monday. I keep asking myself will it actually help? In a way I feel it's self-indulgent of me, committing to three weeks in St Vincent's when I have a daughter who needs me at home. But I know important questions will be asked and it is a good time for self reflection about how I am truly coping – or not coping!

Every day feels like a battle to see who will win: some days I am stronger and I don't let it get me down, other days I feel helpless, sad, depressed. I now know staying in bed actually doesn't help.

The nurse just came in to fill in the chart and asked, 'What would you rate your level of pain as?'

I am sick of rating pain!

Imagine if someone came into any emergency room with obvious burns on their body – they would be treated immediately, they wouldn't be doubted about the severity of their pain. Would someone say to them, 'Between one and ten how would you rate your burns?' And if they said eight or nine would the response be, 'Really, eight or nine? That's quite high, ten being the highest. Are you really at eight or nine? Is the pain really that severe?'

I can say with certainty that they wouldn't have to justify their

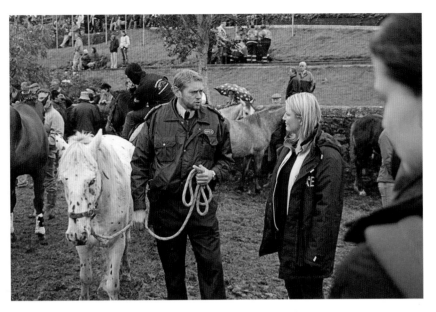

Chief ISPCA Inspector Conor Dowling at the Ballinasloe Fair in 2011 dealing with an abandoned horse.

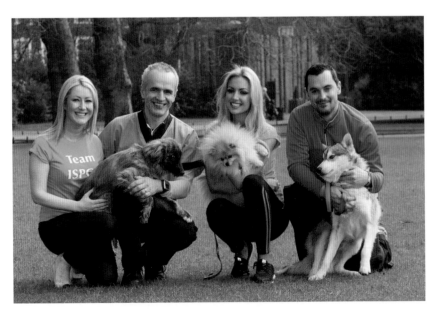

Woman's Mini Marathon photocall for the ISPCA with Pete The Vet, Rosanna Davison and Karl Henry in 2013.
(*Picture by Colm Mahady/Fennells, courtesy of Fennell Photography*)

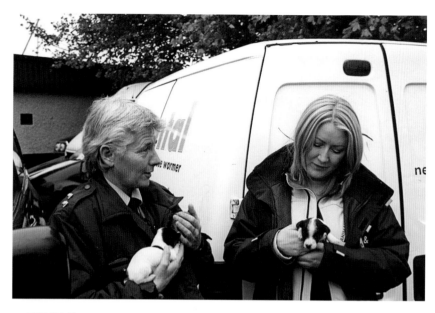

ISPCA Inspector Lisa O'Donovan responding to an allegation of puppies that are for sale too young, during filming for *Animal A&E*.

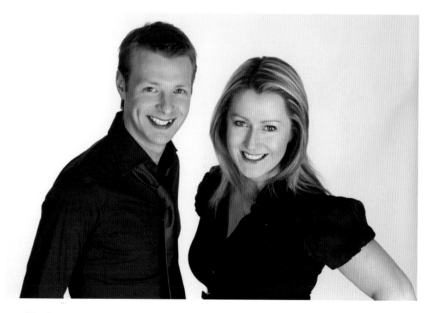

The beginning of a great friendship, *Daytime* on TV3 with Conor Clear. (*Courtesy of Jenny McCarty, photosbyjen*)

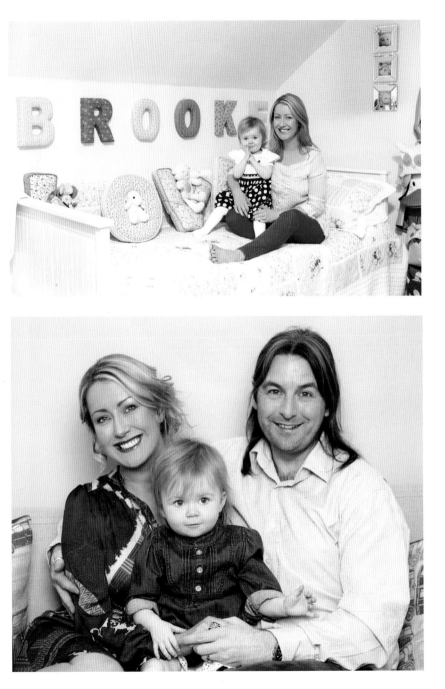

Me with Brooke and David during a VIP shoot in February 2013.
(*Courtesy of Naomi Gaffey*)

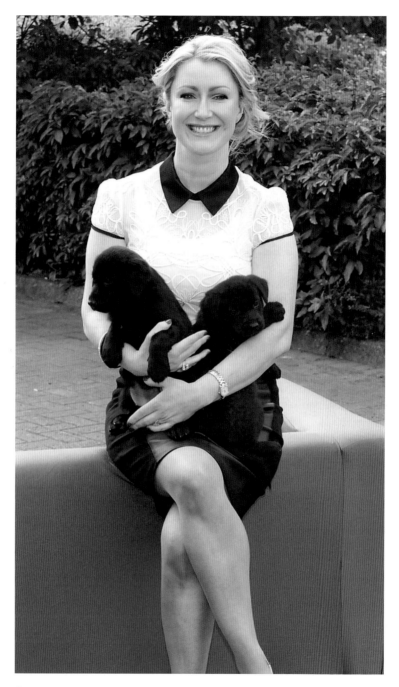

Smiling through a lot of pain at the TV3 autumn launch in August 2013.
(*Courtesy of Brian McEvoy*)

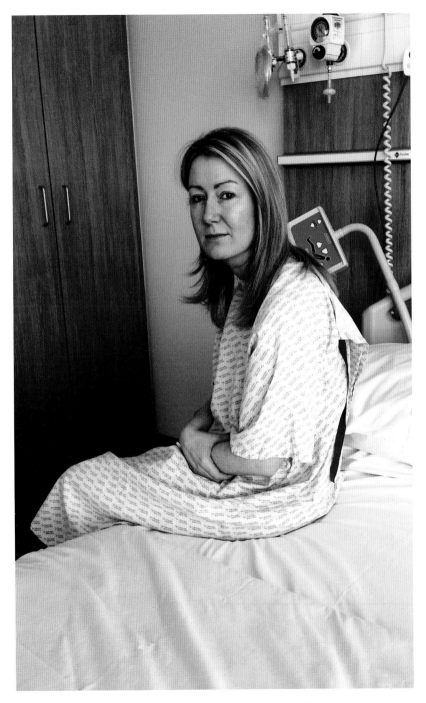

St Vincent's Day Care, December 2013.

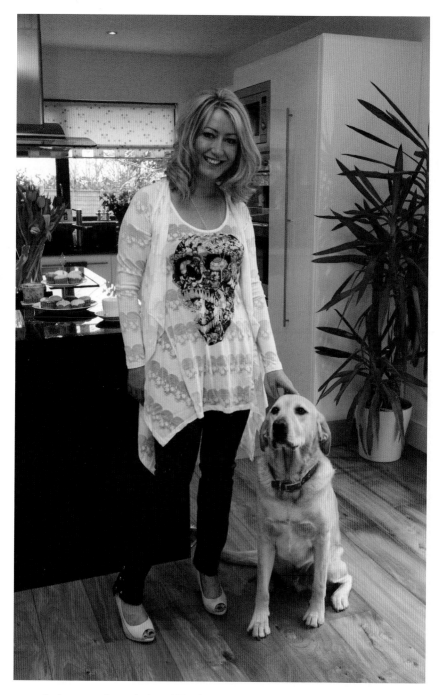

At home with my beloved Dash in May 2012 during an RSVP shoot.
(*Courtesy of Jill O'Meara, www.jillomeara.ie*)

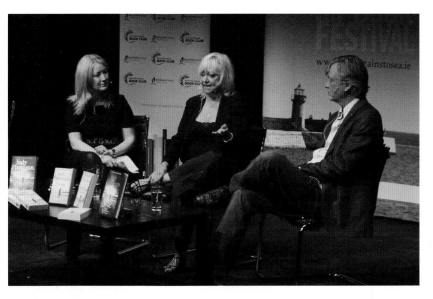

Straight from hospital to the Mountains to Sea dlr Book Festival to interview Richard and Judy in September 2013.
(*Courtesy of Ger Holland Photography*)

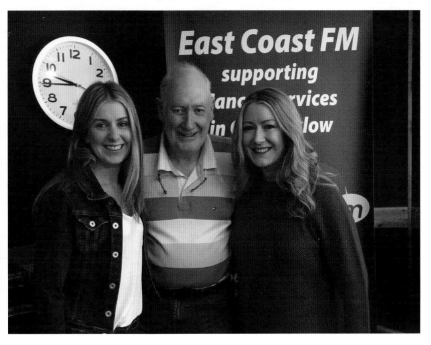

East Coast FM *Morning Show* producer Claire Darmody and presenter Declan Meehan with myself in studio in August 2015.

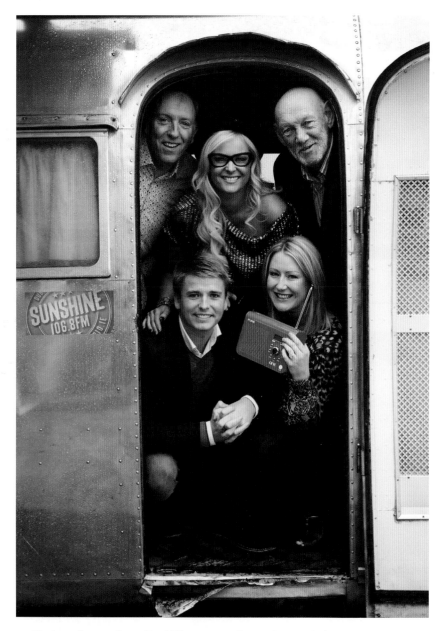

Feeling the sunshine: Paul Harrington, Brian Ormond, Amanda Brunker, Paddy Cole and myself at the Sunshine 106.8 new schedule launch in November 2011.

pain rating, and rightly so. If someone is in pain they are in pain; even if it is not visible it doesn't mean it doesn't exist.

It's not fair, puddles of pity are streaming down my face now.

Please God help the pain to go away. I need to stop this yo-yoing of pain.

The second pain management course marked another significant shift in my life. Once again I wanted to stay on my medication while it was needed, but with the ultimate aim of coming off it, or at least some of it. Without a doubt medication has a very important place in the whole pain-management plan. But relying on medication alone, without addressing how lifestyle changes can help you manage better, is dangerous, for me anyway. I must admit that this time, while I was in a better place to do the pain management course, I wasn't ready to really do the work. Perhaps as a busy working mum I didn't really have a lot of spare time – after all, I was doing the best I could and trying to juggle everything.

So unlike the first pain management course, when I had stopped having my various procedures in St Vincent's, this time I continued getting treatments with Dr Murphy and his team, as I felt they helped me manage the pain and allowed me to continue with my home and work commitments.

Over the months that followed, I was in and out with the team and Dr Murphy concentrated largely on the top half of my back. I had become acutely aware of weakness in my right arm and hand. It was becoming quite apparent that something wasn't right; I had neck, shoulder and elbow pain, and the pain down my arm became a constant part of my everyday pain. For me, when a new area of pain starts to persist, I get worried that the pain is somehow spreading. I wanted to explore what might be causing this arm pain.

15

The Year that Broke
the Camel's Back

I started 2013 as I start every new year, full of positivity and praying that this would be the year when I finally got on top of the pain.

In early January I made an appointment to see Dr Bleakley and we spoke some more about my work and the way I was juggling everything. She quickly pointed out that I still hadn't fully embraced the principle of 'acceptance'. In a very supportive manner she suggested, 'Perhaps you should think about telling more people about your problems, especially in work – they could help you pace and space your activities. Telling more friends and family members would also be positive, as they might be able to offer support with Brooke.' We also introduced a new tablet to see if it could help with my increased upper body pain, and upped the dosage of my current tablets to help with sleep.

When I left her office I thought a lot about what she had said. As a result I decided to set some ground rules about my availability for the new series of *Animal A&E* that I was about to start shooting. On each new series a new producer and filming crew are appointed, so I had a chat with my new producer and explained that I could physically only do one or maybe two days' shooting per week, as I had to factor in the impact the long journeys and even longer filming days had on my health.

I was nervous broaching the subject, and initially it didn't go down very well. He scheduled a meeting with the executive producer, Andy, to talk about the schedule. Luckily I had worked with Andy since the very first series, and he had become a good friend and confidant, who knew about my chronic pain. In the meeting we had a long discussion about spacing out our shoot days. Often we would leave Dublin very early to travel to various destinations around the country, film for a full day and then have the long car journey back to Ballymount and into TV3 to wrap up any clerical details from the day's shoot, so it was a demanding gig for everyone. I managed to convince the new producer that both himself and the crew would thank me in a few weeks for having only one long rescue day a week. I assured them both I was as committed as ever to this fifth series, and, after all, I was also the associate producer, so I had no intention of letting them down. Naturally, if we needed to add in an extra day for a breaking rescue case I would. In fairness my new producer was very good about it once he could see I wasn't being a diva but, instead of explaining the extent of my 'back issues', I just left it at that and we all got on with it.

I started to think a lot about the whole concept of accepting chronic pain, talking about it more openly, maybe even publicly in the media. I decided to embrace chronic pain as part of who I am and, without telling anyone, I wrote an article about my experience with chronic pain and submitted it to *Woman's Way*. The lovely editor, Áine Toner, liked it and miraculously agreed to publish it. I was a nervous wreck because this was, for me, in many respects a very brave step – admitting in a public forum the struggles I faced dealing with persistent pain.

I was shocked and totally overwhelmed by the feedback. People from all over Ireland reached out to me through Facebook to share their stories, and it felt wonderful to have it out in the open finally. I went on to talk about it on *Midday* and in various newspaper articles later that year. Having the article published really empowered me to have the courage to finally share my secret struggle.

Now that my secret was out, I felt that people were somehow looking at me more closely to see if they could spot the pain, and sometimes I felt that certain people questioned whether the pain really existed. I was getting offers to do many different types of work, in addition to my weekly radio show and TV projects. For the most part they were small MC presenting roles or charity work and I enjoyed it, but the extra hours, coupled with family life and pain, meant I wasn't pacing myself well and my busy schedule left little time for anything else.

As the year continued and work commitments increased, my pain was growing to worrying levels. I tried to keep perspective by writing in my journal, but while outwardly I seemed to be coping well, behind my smiles for the cameras I was struggling. A few different work events came up that proved all the extra work was pushing me to breaking point.

March 2013

Give me strength.

I always feel pretty useless around this time of the year, leading up to the mini marathon – every year I hope that this will be the year that I am able to complete it. I was asked to do it for the ISPCA, which is so dear to my heart and I would love to do it. We had the photo-shoot today in St Stephen's Green with Pete Wedderburn, Rosanna Davison and Karl Henry asking people to join Team ISPCA, and naturally they want me to sign up. In my brain I am thinking, I think I can do this, and I still believe I will, but just not this year.

I should have been forthcoming about why I couldn't commit to it. I think sometimes it's the old issue again of looking so well on the outside. So raising it with someone feels like you're an attention-seeker or a moaner. And I can understand why it is tough for people to see me and think of course you can do it, walk it.

Anyway, I feel really crap about it, I am wondering should I just do it – I keep thinking is it fear avoidance?

I did sign up a few years back but then I stepped out of training because of a bad flare-up. The reaction I got still haunts me. I truly felt like a big loser, and to be told that women in their eighties can do it didn't help matters, it just made me beat myself up for having this pain and for not feeling physically strong enough to push through. I think if there was a year where I hadn't much on and I could build up strength for a number of months beforehand I could do it. This year, I am just trying to cope as best I can and already I am really working through the pain, really forcing myself to get on with whatever job I have to do. I was in a lot of pain even through the photo-shoot. A x

In May of that year my good friend Valerie Roe asked me to MC an event, 'Strictly for Soccer', along with FAI Chief Executive John Delaney. We had a brief run-through and all seemed well. However, when the house lights went down, the back of the stage area went completely black and when I was walking off I couldn't see the exit. I had a relatively minor misstep coming down from the stage and both John and I fell down a couple of feet. It wasn't a fall to the floor as John managed to grab hold of me, but I knew instantly that whatever way I had twisted my body wasn't good. Within minutes I felt my back going into spasm. For anyone else it might not have even registered, but for someone with back weakness and constant pain, it certainly didn't help matters.

I reached for my constant companion, pain-relief medication, and took as much as I could to get through the rest of the evening. This little setback started a cycle of increased pain and when I mentioned it to Dr Murphy, he said it was possible I had whiplash from the incident. He helped to get the pain under control and we did a number of pain procedures to try to alleviate the pain.

By then I was on another combination of medications with Dr Bleakley, which seemed okay. I was functioning and coping, but there was one particular medication that I felt was having more adverse effects than good. It left me feeling a little spacey, slower, lethargic, and it seemed to affect my cognitive responses. Over time the medication had definitely affected my personality, sex drive, metabolism and, of course, my weight, although the effects had built up slowly.

I had hoped to come off one of my newer tablets completely and reduce others, but I hadn't yet returned to Dr Bleakley to talk it through with her. As the weeks passed I was getting busier and busier with work and I suppose because I was freelance I was telling myself to take the work while I was being offered it, thinking that the next month would be quiet. But the lull I was hoping for never happened. It was great to be in demand but it meant putting my medication concerns on the back burner until I made a stupid and potentially dangerous decision.

In June 2013 I was asked to cover Declan Meehan's mid-morning talk show on East Coast FM for two weeks. I was thrilled and gladly accepted. I loved working with the team, all of whom I knew very well, and it's a great show – a mix of light entertainment and breaking news, plus local issues. With the regular presenter away I would be able to skew it in a different way, make it lighter, with topics like parenting, fashion, TV, etc. – nothing too taxing – and I thought that during the summer months there is never much breaking news anyway. Famous last words!

The Monday I started, probably the biggest news item of the year broke. Astonishing tape recordings from inside Anglo-Irish Bank were broadcast. The recordings of telephone conversations revealed for the first time how the bank's top executives had lied to the government about the true extent of losses at the institution. The scandal was a massive story and we had Paul Williams, the reporter who broke the story, live on air. It was a complex banking story that required measured questions to peel away the many layers of the scandal to highlight for the listeners what it meant for the man and woman on the street. It was out of my comfort zone, but I had great support from a wonderful producer and I loved the challenge.

In the days that followed, as many more recordings were leaked, the story took centre stage. Then, in addition to the Anglo tapes, another massive political story broke. It was revealed that four TDs lost the party whip after voting against the Protection of Life During Pregnancy Bill. One of the 'rogue' TDs, as they were being called in the media, was Billy Timmins, a local Wicklow representative, so we got an exclusive interview with the man himself.

With such monumental stories expected to run for the coming days I wanted to feel sharper and more alert, so I decided to stop taking one of my tablets, which I believed was contributing to my feeling of fogginess, as well as an irritating dry mouth. Of course I should have consulted my doctor, as I was soon to discover.

Initially, I didn't feel much sharper, but I was off the tablets and I felt more in control. In my second week we had another exclusive interview. There was local interest in a distressed property auction taking place in the Shelbourne Hotel in Dublin, and we had pre-arranged a call from inside the auction room with a lady who would give us an update on some properties in

Wicklow that our listeners were familiar with. We contacted her, as agreed, for the interview, but seconds before we went live, an angry mob of protestors stampeded the venue. By a stroke of luck we heard the story unfold live on air. A tense scene played out as gardaí tried to calm the situation. It was wonderful content for live radio.

The following day, against the odds, another massive story broke! When I went into the studio for the pre-show chat, the wonderful producer Claire Darmody said, 'BOD hasn't been picked! We have a live link to Australia.' To my shame, in my sporting ignorance I didn't know who or what BOD stood for. I needed to get the back story quickly and ask the right questions before we went live.

Of course, the BOD in question was Ireland's national rugby team captain, Brian O'Driscoll, generally considered the finest player of his generation. He had just been sensationally dropped from the British and Irish Lions team to play in the final test match against Australia, with the three-match test series hanging in the balance. O'Driscoll was the darling of Irish sport. This tour was his swansong with the Lions – he had already signalled his intention to retire from the sport. And to add a little spice, the coach who had dropped him had once been the Ireland national rugby coach, and some said he was still bitter about how he had been sacked out of the blue by the IRFU.

So it was a sensational sporting story in its own right, and once again we had a Wicklow local, former Irish rugby international Shane Byrne, in Australia filling us in on the breaking story. The texts were coming in quick and fast.

As my second week drew to a close I was feeling anxious and a little strange, which I put down to being challenged and out of my comfort zone. This feeling was steadily building and I had never, ever felt this way before, so I was unsure of what it was. Although I was really enjoying the radio show and everyone else was happy with me, I felt I was out of my depth at times. I was getting some great compliments on my handling of the stories and the producer, Claire, was happy (and she is very honest), so this was mostly an internal feeling. On the last day I went in feeling tired, shaky, out of sorts and just not myself. I hadn't slept well the night before, so I put it down to that. With hindsight I know what was happening, but at the time I didn't even consider that stopping my medication – cold turkey – could be linked to the sort of uncomfortable feelings I was experiencing.

One of the team had baked some lovely cupcakes to mark my last day, so we all tucked in during our morning chat about what was ahead on the show. Luckily, it was a little bit more relaxed than recent days as Paul Connolly, a colleague of mine from TV3, was coming in for an extended Friday interview. As the show started I realised I had a very dry mouth. It was a common side effect of the meds I had been taking, but it can also sometimes happen when you're nervous. I thought to myself, 'You're not nervous, this is easy peasy to you, Andrea.' Yet I couldn't get rid of the dryness and I felt I could hear a 'click' in my voice; again, this is not very unusual – I thought I just needed to warm up my vocal cords during the first ad break. I carry throat spray if I am on air, so I used some spray, just in case it was the beginning of a sore throat. But it felt as though something wasn't right in my throat and whatever it was seemed to be getting worse.

The next hour is a virtual blank. I felt out of control, I was constantly asking for water, the team were checking if I was all right and I was saying I didn't feel well, and all the while we had a talk radio show going out live on air. I was a mess. I think I managed to pull it off, but at one point I wanted to just walk out. When we went to the news bulletin I said to the producer, 'I don't feel well, I think I'm allergic to something, I can't swallow, my lips are tingling and I think I'm having a heart attack, I can't really breathe.'

She was shell-shocked. I could tell she was genuinely worried, but time is not on your side when your show is live, and my TV3 colleague was already in the studio. I went in and told him I felt 'weird', apologised and said, 'Just keep talking.' We started the interview and he was a true pro, talking nineteen to the dozen. To any listeners it would have sounded perfectly normal. We kept Paul a little longer than we had planned, then had some live music at the end of the hour. To pad it out my producer actually came into the studio and did a super TV slot – she could see that I was definitely not right. That was my worst ever experience on radio or TV. Just writing about it now is bringing it all back; it was one of the scariest things I have ever gone through.

When we came off air, I apologised to the producer and said I had to go. I got into my car and drove for five minutes, when I ran into some minor roadworks with a stop–go system in operation. There was a small build-up of traffic and while I was waiting, I thought, 'I am going to die in this car.' I thought I had been poisoned by one of the cupcakes we had eaten that morning, so clearly I had lost all rational thought! In a panic, I did a dangerous manoeuvre, turned the car around and drove like a madwoman back to the station, where I asked the producer to call an ambulance! She rang my husband, who told me to call my doctor and thankfully my amazing GP took my call immediately. I explained everything and she said it sounded as though I was experiencing a panic/anxiety attack. When she asked if I had changed my meds recently, or taken anything new, I explained that I had stopped taking one of the tablets. She told me that I shouldn't have just come off it completely: 'You have to come off gradually, reducing the dose slowly.' She faxed a prescription for some relaxants to a local chemist and I took them straight away.

I was shaken, embarrassed and still feeling that I was having an out-of-body experience, but at least I knew I wasn't going to die and that the relaxants would kick in. That was my first, and only, panic attack, but it gave me the greatest sympathy for anyone who suffers from these – mine was horrifyingly scary and something I never wish to revisit. Over the weekend I had a few milder incidences, but now that I knew what was causing it, I was okay.

However, the whole experience had a profound effect on me. It left me almost afraid to work and I cancelled my diary for the next few weeks.

August 2013

The last few weeks have been almost surreal. I haven't been able to write in a while as I really felt like I was having some sort of break-down. It has been a really difficult few weeks. I have managed now to get completely off the dreaded tablet I had elected just to stop taking, cold turkey! What was I thinking? I had to go back on them and come off them slowly. Penny has been great, I am so lucky she is my GP. It has not been easy, in fact the most difficult weeks in recent years, mak-ing sense of the panic attack and then being almost terrified it might happen again.

I can't begin to explain how hard it was. Afterwards I felt really depressed, anxious and exhausted. It is scary, feeling almost like you are looking at yourself and not even recognising who you are. I was so down on myself, really hard on myself. I had to take some time off work, I found myself not able to come out of my bedroom, I was so scared, fearful, hopeless. I was so sad. I suppose the hardest thing for me was feeling out of control for the two weeks I had to cancel seeing people.

Since yesterday, I feel like I have turned a corner mentally and now, looking back at the last few weeks, I can't even imagine it was me, the hopelessness I felt – it seems almost unimaginable that was me. I feel proud of myself that I managed to come off the meds.

I now have a huge respect and admiration for anyone who has anxiety attacks, it's crazy to think that something so scary can manifest from not taking tablets. A x

Some positives did come out of the panic attack – I had a better understanding about the importance of taking my medication regularly and not self-medicating or mixing any tablets without advice from a healthcare specialist. Penny also suggested I start going to the same chemist every month to fill my prescription so I could build up a relationship with them in case I needed to get an urgent prescription faxed over in the future. Before then I would stop at any random chemist so I had no set pharmacy. I took her advice and I now know all the team at Lloyds in Shankhill; they keep my prescription on file and remind me when it needs to be updated.

I left the memory of my panic attack behind me and by September I was once again getting lots of exciting work offers. I was getting good relief from the procedures with Dr Murphy, which was amazing. Sometimes I would go in for a procedure with the intention of getting my neck zapped but my coccyx area might become more painful, and I would have a chat and say, 'I need to do this area, Dr Murphy.' He was very flexible. And while my pain didn't disappear, I felt that either my expectations had changed or the procedures had advanced, but I could really feel the benefit, particularly around the neck, shoulders and upper back area.

When my pain is under control I am like a different person. After a successful procedure I feel as though someone has plugged me in, my battery is charged and I am ready to go. I feel positive, I'm creative, I have great work ideas and plans. I want to plan holidays, dinners with friends, play dates with Brooke. Life is better than good. Life is amazing. When I feel like this I am joyous, almost pain free and feel invincible. I find myself singing, 'I'm on the top of the world'. I feel like calling Dr Murphy's secretary to say 'I'm cured'.

Sadly this lovely utopia doesn't always last too long. Oftentimes I slightly overdo it, I am little over-zealous, but I just feel so happy when there is a big reduction in the pain. During these times I generally start booking up my work diary, confident this feeling will linger. The very strange thing about pain is that you can feel great today and in crippling pain tomorrow; it isn't predictable and I think that is the bit I struggle with most. I truly do try to take the advice of my doctors and pace myself workwise, and space activities, but sadly when I commit to doing a gig, I can't really predict how my pain will be. I try to only commit to jobs I really want to be part of, so I do say no a lot. It seems almost impossible to juggle work with chronic pain.

I now know what my GP Penny meant about acceptance – part of that is being able to tell people, 'I have chronic pain, there is a chance this could flare up and I may not be able to fulfil my work commitments.' But the reality is that I don't think anyone would hire me if I were that honest. I also hate letting people down, so occasionally after a day procedure and totally against doctor's orders, I would go in to work and try to grin and bear it. Then, in late September 2013, something happened that made me realise this would have to stop.

The Mountains to Sea dlr Book Festival is a wonderful

celebration of writing and it takes place each year in Dún Laoghaire. That September television presenter and author Judy Finnigan was the special guest at the festival. She was there to talk about her first novel, *Eloise*. A week before the event the scheduled presenter had to pull out and I was asked to fill in. When I agreed I wasn't planning for pain, in fact I was feeling good, but I had been having intermittent problems with my neck and arm and without warning it went into spasm. I called Dr Murphy's secretary and she booked me in for a PRF in the first available appointment, which was on Friday morning. As a frequent day patient I knew the drill; being the first in theatre meant the procedure would be over early. I had to eat my tea and toast, go to the toilet and if all was well I'd be discharged. The PRF went well but afterwards I was groggier and in more post-procedure pain than normal. I slept after the procedure, which was totally unusual for me, and awoke feeling awful. I got some pain relief and rested some more. Even though I felt exhausted and in pain I had to get home and get ready for the early evening event. With great discomfort I managed to get up and my husband drove me home; shortly afterwards he drove me to the event. I felt a little spacey but I got on with it.

When I got to the theatre I met with the organisers, who told me that Judy was feeling very ill. There was a possibility she wasn't going to be able to do the talk and Richard, her husband, might have to do it. If she was feeling strong enough to go on, Richard would sit on stage as well in case she had to leave. This was perfect, as I was sure the audience would be only too delighted to see the famous TV couple Richard and Judy. I was excited about the chat, as I loved her book and had lots of questions to ask her.

We met briefly before we went on stage. 'I'm so sorry,' she said, 'I'm feeling very poorly and I just don't know if I'll be able to go on stage.' She was very pale and it was obvious she was in discomfort. 'Don't worry,' I replied. 'Do whatever you need to.' Then she saw my neck plaster and asked what had happened. I explained, 'I was in hospital earlier today and had a procedure for a chronic pain problem, so I'm feeling out of sorts myself – maybe neither of us will make it on!' We both laughed and began to chat about a mutual friend in the world of TV.

When the time came she decided to go on with Richard by her side. The evening was a great success and they were both wonderfully interesting people to interview – warm, engaging, professional – and the audience and I enjoyed listening to them enormously. We spoke briefly afterwards and I thanked them both and asked Judy how she was feeling. 'Not much better,' she replied.

'No one in the audience would have noticed, you sailed through the conversation with a smile. I hope you make a speedy recovery.' Then we said our goodbyes and she left.

The chat once again really highlighted to me that you just never know what is going on behind the scenes when you meet people, and the saying, 'Never judge a book by its cover' came to mind.

I suppose after that night I realised the duality of my life. Was I an eccedentesiast, hiding my pain with a smile? There and then, I made a decision to be more forthcoming about my pain. I did an interview with one of the national newspapers and for the first time I was honest about the realities of living in chronic pain. For me this was a brave move and a bit of a gamble. Unlike the *Woman's Way* article, which I wrote myself, I was relying now on a journalist's interpretation. So often in the media things can be reported out of context, so I was opening myself up to be judged about my secret pain and felt very vulnerable.

Pain-*free* Life

In the name of pain

I was out last night at my friend T's house and she was asking how I was doing. Since the newspaper article about my chronic pain and my health, everyone is asking me 'How is the back?' 'What happened to the back?' I am getting countless offers from different people who can work wonders with back complaints, so in some ways being open and honest about my back is a bit of a hindrance, as I am constantly having to explain myself. It was way easier when I could just put on a smiley face and ignore it.

I found myself having that exact conversation last night in a friend's house. She was introducing me to a friend of hers and was explaining about my back pain, which opened up the conversation about me and my condition and the various magic cures that could 'fix' me. So I began to explain – as we often find ourselves doing – that unless you have experienced chronic pain it is so difficult to understand that someone who is sitting in front of you, looking fine and healthy, is in pain.

I got the sceptical look from my friend's friend – who I'd just met. Then T, trying to almost validate me to her friend, said, 'Andrea has a real problem. She isn't like all those people who say, I have a pain here, there and everywhere all in your head shit. What do they call that? Fibromyalgia?' (Even writing this now I am so annoyed with that statement.)

Last night I found myself getting really angry, saying to them, 'It's not all in people's heads. Do you really think people want to have this, want to be judged, asked if the pain is a figment of their imagination?' I was so annoyed that they judged a certain group of people because of the name of their condition. 'I happen to know so many people who have that and I see how they suffer, often in silence, daily. I haven't been diagnosed with fibromyalgia but the name isn't important to me, I don't care what condition, label, or whatever people want to call it, but, for some reason, for me and many others our pain gate has been opened and, for a reason we don't fully know, our body is in pain. That's not the symptom. That is the disease. The pain is the disease.'

My outburst surprised them both and we went on to talk about it and how I felt everyone just dismisses it. Even for me, someone who has had two successful TV shows, when I pitched my idea for a documentary on pain, no one was interested. It broke my heart that others didn't believe in the idea. Someone said it would be difficult to actually portray, as we can't really tell if people are really in pain. It wouldn't make good telly! The list of negatives goes on.

I just got so upset again last night relating the story to them, as that rejection really hurt me. That's what having pain disciplines you to accept: rejection! No one believes you, no one can fully explain why! From doctor to doctor, specialist to specialist, and oftentimes you are just left asking, 'Why me? Why do I have this mysterious pain?'

My friend for the first time got a little insight into my world managing pain. She said, 'So are you in pain now?' I said, 'Yes. Sitting is a pain in the ass!' We laughed. She said, 'I am trying to get my head around you being in pain. Why can't you just take a tablet or get something done to fix it?'

Well, if we had the answer to that we would all be very rich.

Then to my surprise, she got her work hat on and we started to debate and discuss the whole concept of perceptions of pain and living with pain. Both of them worked in the marketing and branding business for many years and they agreed that pain needed to be portrayed in the right way, and people with fibromyalgia, to her mind at least, just seemed moaney!

She was being really honest and I had to respect her for that, but it did make me think. Maybe nobody believed in my idea for a documentary about pain because I was selling it wrong. Could we package pain better so the world could understand its complexity? Could we sell it in such a way that society would stop judging others who have it and start to see the truth of what it is like to live in pain every day, constantly? Instead of looking at these people as 'moaney' we should salute them for being strong, brave, resilient – they are the champions of chronic pain. I thought to myself, the world needs to see pain and chronic pain differently. Maybe she is right, pain needs a marketing makeover!

16

Surprising Results

For most of 2013 I was generally happy with how I was managing the pain, although it meant taking a lot of tablets and regularly having a number of procedures. If I could sort out the arm and hand weakness, that would settle my mind. I mentioned it to Dr Murphy and he decided to get some nerve conduction tests done.

The tests were done in hospital. They hooked me up to a pretty cool-looking device; if I knew what a lie detector looked like I imagine they would be quite similar. The device has a scale to measure your nerve pulses while tiny electric shocks are used to stimulate the nerves in your hand, wrist and elbow. It made sense to me that it could be a nerve issue and I didn't really expect it to be anything else. For me the weakness was more worrying than the pain, so I was keen to get an answer to this new and niggling problem.

Dr Murphy said that everything looked normal enough, so he now wanted to get scans done again. It had been a while since I had had any scans – it was definitely pre-pregnancy – and this time I had a number of upper body MRIs, which I hadn't had before because my pain had largely been confined to my lower back.

I went for my scans in November. They took a little over an hour. You are wheeled into a tunnel, which is pretty strange in itself, although I had been in one many times, and normally you can listen to music to hide the strange noise of the machine, but on that morning my mind was focused on how I was going to juggle a really busy time workwise. It was just before Christmas and I was in pre-production for an airport show; I was finishing another series of *Animal A&E*; I had committed myself to my annual December stint on a charity radio station, Christmas FM; and there was my own radio show, of course. With so much going on, I knew I would be overdoing things.

I thought that if I could just find the energy to get through December, the new year would bring more balance, and I could address my pain then, so I decided to just take whatever medication I could to keep the pain at a controllable level. After having the MRI scans I put them out of my head; I didn't really think that the scan results would shed any real light on my current pain situation. How wrong I was.

My doctor rang me at work one morning at the start of December. He wanted to talk to me about the results of the recent MRI scans and explained that he wanted to call me to let me know before the letter arrived with the findings. He also mentioned something called Chiari malformation 1. I had never heard of it before, but my scan showed that I had it. I was going to be in hospital on Friday for another procedure, so we could chat more about it then.

When we spoke on Friday he suggested I see a surgeon, Mr Poynton at the Mater, for his opinion on surgery options for some disc degeneration in my cervical and thoracic area. Mr Poynton would also be able to advise on surgical options for the Chiari malformation.

At the time I wasn't really thinking much further than the next few weeks. I needed pain relief to see me through December, but once I had completed my work commitments I could slow things down in the new year and explore this new diagnosis. I parked the Chiari malformation diagnosis as something to be dealt with at a later stage.

At the same time, I realised that my life was becoming a bit overwhelming; I was managing the pain, the tablets and my workload, and now I had a new diagnosis to factor into the mix. I knew deep down what I needed to do. What I did next wasn't planned and it was almost a spur of the moment decision. I asked my line manager in TV3 for some leave in the new year. It was a strange move, which surprised many of my colleagues. I wasn't unhappy, and I was probably busier than ever – I had recently been asked to cover presenting *Midday* and I had my own successful TV shows – so workwise I couldn't have wished for more. However, I followed my gut instinct and it was done – I was given three months' leave from January.

It was definitely the silly season at work. December passed by so quickly and for the most part I didn't think about Chiari malformation 1, or even tell any friends about this new development. I was working away on TV programmes and radio shows, being my usual positive self, looking forward to Christmas and trying to push through the pain.

Very quickly after 25 December my mind shifted and I was ready to tackle Chiari. First things first: to research what Chiari is and what it means to have a malformation score of 1. Of course I found a lot of websites with many scary facts, but it did seem that this could be the cause of some of my mystery pain and maybe even my hearing problems as a child. I found myself reading an awful lot about Chiari and what follows are some of the basic facts which I discovered on the websites of the National Institute of Neurological Disorders and Stroke and the American Syringomyelia and Chiari Alliance Project.

Pain-*free* Life

What is Chiari?

Chiari malformations (CM) are structural defects in the cerebellum. Normally this sits in an indented space at the lower rear of the skull, above the foramen magnum (an opening to the spinal canal). When part of it is located below the foramen magnum, it is called a Chiari malformation.

What are the symptoms?

Some CMs are asymptomatic, but in other cases, individuals complain of neck pain, balance problems, muscle weakness, numbness or other abnormal feelings in the arms or legs, dizziness, vision problems, difficulty swallowing, ringing or buzzing in the ears, hearing loss, vomiting, insomnia, depression, or headaches made worse by coughing or straining. Hand coordination and fine motor skills may also be affected. Symptoms may change, depending on the build-up of cerebrospinal fluid and the resulting pressure on the tissues and nerves.

How is it treated?

For some, medication may ease certain symptoms, such as pain. For functional disturbances or to halt the progression of damage to the central nervous system, surgery is the only current treatment. Many people who have surgery see a reduction in their symptoms and/or prolonged periods of relative stability. More than one surgery may be needed.[1]

Is surgery a cure?

No. Surgery is a treatment, not a cure. Some symptoms are more likely to improve with surgery than others.

1   http://www.ninds.nih.gov/disorders/chiari/detail_chiari.htm

Is Chiari fatal?

Chiari malformation is not typically fatal. However, a CM that extends into the brainstem can affect the breathing and swallowing centres. If these centres are severely affected, there can be a risk of serious complications.[2]

Depressing reading!

I needed to take immediate action and look at the positives. Could this be the cause of all my pain? I felt I needed to seek out an expert who specialised in Chiari. I found very little information about treatment in Ireland, so I started to look further afield and my research led to a doctor who was constantly mentioned for his outstanding work and commitment to treating Chiari patients. He had evaluated and treated several thousand patients from all over the world. I was sold. A neurosurgeon and Chiari specialist, he was based in the Chiari Institute in New York. I needed to see him.

The email I sent to the institute is a vivid snapshot of how worried I was about this strange diagnosis. The message title itself, 'URGENT APPOINTMENT', pretty much summed up my mood. I felt a sudden urgency for everything – the pressure was on in many respects. I had taken time off work, so I needed to make it count. I didn't have any definite plan other than to explore everything and anything that might help with my wellness and my own pain management programme. Mixed with this was the panic of having a rare condition that could be fatal! As always, there was a glimmer of hope that maybe this doctor would finally be the answer to my prayers. I got a message back

2   http://asap.org/index.php/medical-articles/questions-asked-by-the-newly-diagnosed/

within a few days with good news – I had an appointment at the Chiari Institute in New York on 30 January 2014.

By a wonderful coincidence my husband had a work commitment in New York at the end of the month, so I took this as a sign and we made the decision to travel to New York as a family, bringing Brooke and my mam. While I was fortunate enough to get an appointment with a specialist, they couldn't confirm whether I would actually get to speak to the doctor I had read about, but we would talk to a member of his team who could review my scans. I had to fill in a number of long online questionnaires about my medical history and I had to bring all relevant MRI scans. Apart from that I didn't know what to expect or what my diagnosis would be. But I remained positive that January would mark the beginning of my new pain management system at home.

31st December 2013

We had a lovely evening with our friends Kevin and Muriel ringing in the new year! We all took part in a ritual of writing out our goals for 2014 and burying them in their garden in the earth. I think the idea is that our dreams will grow in the soil like little seeds, and blossom in 2014. Then we had to write down things we wish to leave behind in 2013 and we burned them in a little bonfire in the garden! It was immensely good fun and quite liberating. Interestingly when I wrote down what I don't want, one word was scribbled, almost without thinking. I wrote 'PAIN', I don't want pain! So my mission is to somehow try to remove pain from my day-to-day life.

It has really inspired me to really get focused on what I want to achieve in the next three months and for the year ahead. I had a jolt of determination this evening after I wrote down my health goals. There is something so powerful in taking the time to actually write down how we feel and what we want to achieve. I was reminded just how important it is for me to write daily, so I am starting now with my new health mission for 2014.

My new health mission:

I am working on my wellness and I now embark on an important health mission for myself. I realise that I need to participate in daily relaxation activities. I will commit to my wellness plan of writing in my journal honestly, counting my blessings, daily walks, eating healthy food and living in the best way for me.

I need to avoid stress and deal with the stress I can't avoid in a gentle way. 'Gentle' is my new word for pacing. I want to live and treat myself in a gentle way. I want to take optimum care of my body physically, emotionally and spiritually; this is my priority now.

I know and accept no single thing, or pill, can help cure my chronic pain but I am healing myself the best way I know how.

I hope to live a full and pain-free life in 2014.

Blessings & abundance, Andrea x

17

New Year, New Wellness Plan

Taking the time out to get well was the best decision for me and I wanted to get as well as I could be. I had three months' leave from my TV3 work, and I wasn't taking on any new work. I had decided to continue with my Saturday morning radio show but from Monday to Friday, while Brooke was at Montessori, my focus was on taking care of my health, even though I didn't really have a concrete plan on 1 January 2014.

I wanted to reduce my medication, I knew that much. I also promised myself that for the next three months I would write in my journal every day. I had started doing this during my first pain management course, and later I kept a gratitude diary, but I wasn't writing religiously every day. I decided that I would document truthfully how I was feeling. I needed to be open and honest about my experiences and my successes and failures along this road, especially if I was going to come off the medication. This decision proved right and it served as a great road map later when I needed to journey back and remind myself exactly how I had been feeling and the subsequent lessons I had learned.

Taking the time off work to focus fully on my wellness was all about me taking control of my life and my health. With time to reflect, I made a firm decision to detox all areas of my life. I wanted to remove any limiting influences on my health and well-being. I made a decision to take notice of my thoughts, catching myself when fear-based thoughts brought down my mood. I needed to stay positive and I wanted to believe that I could manifest change in my body and heal myself. I could see that I needed to get some balance in my life. I wrote healing affirmations every day. I wanted to read books on healing and fill my mind with positive stories of people who had healed their lives, in the hope that I could too.

Friday 3rd January 2014

Good morning first Friday of 2014, I only wrote affirmations yester-day so today is the official start of the wellness journal!

Happy New Year, but sadly not a new start to my day. It was a typical start, with another pretty-much sleepless night. I woke up in so much pain, feeling uncomfortable, looked at my phone every hour, watching time pass, I coaxed myself back to sleep, but the time edged ever closer to my wake-up time.

I find that, even though I am awake, I have that 'medication hangover' from the tablets, so while I am technically awake, I have no energy or will to move. I'm kind of groggy – both mentally and physically – so this morning I just decided to force myself out of bed to write in my journal, rather than let the constant clutter of thoughts race around in my head.

I went into a church yesterday and picked up Our Lady of Lourdes Novena. I've just read it. I will try to continue it for the next few days. I prayed for good health for me, for my family and for all my pain friends.

I seem to pray a lot about pain, or being pain free. I had a chat yesterday with a good friend, Audrey. She was talking about her deep concerns about money, bills, pressure with work, and asked me to say a prayer for her – she was tired of worrying about money. I promised I would pray for abundance and pennies from heaven. I said honestly to her, 'Don't worry about money, it will come, it's only paper, it's only energy, don't worry too much.'

She then said to me, 'Everyone is the same, we all have money worries' and I said in an honest, matter-of-fact way, 'I don't worry about money.' She seemed a bit shocked and she asked me, 'So, Andrea, what do you worry about?'

I thought for a moment and said my health, mostly my pain, and it really surprised her. She went very quiet after that. And since yesterday I can't stop thinking about the conversation, especially as I have decided to take three months off work to get my health and pain better. Maybe I should worry more about money and where it will come from!

It's hard to admit that the pain in recent months has affected my life so badly. I feel I can't work, or feel overwhelmed trying to manage everything with the undercurrent of pain constantly crashing around everything. While I sit here in the silence of the morning, alone with my thoughts, I wonder what it would be like not to live with pain, would I worry about different things? Every day I worry in some way about pain. No matter what I do, I have to include pain in my plans. As I look out of the window to the sky and the clouds, I wonder how it would feel to be light like the clouds. I seem to carry this heaviness around with me. Maybe other people don't have the feeling of being ground down, but I feel this pressure – sometimes the pain in my head, neck, back feels like it is literally pushing me down.

I am feeling particularly down this morning. Maybe in truth I do worry about money, and the fact that I am not working looms bigger than I would like to admit?

I suppose, in the months leading up to my decision to leave work, I was becoming more tangled in a web of lies. I wasn't coping, I wasn't happy, I wasn't pacing and I wasn't looking to myself for the answers to my own recovery. In the weeks and months leading up to my decision, I was desperately trying to live. I would drag myself out of bed in the morning, get my daughter ready for crèche, go to work and have great difficulty carrying out my normal tasks like using a computer, my voice-over booth, or being out on film shoots. Everything was a massive chore. I put so much energy into pushing myself through the day, desperately popping another pill to suppress the pain and all the while really causing more stress in my body and general unease in my body and my life. I wasn't feeling in control of anything, every day was like groundhog day, I felt powerless. So I feel in some way I had no choice. I need this time to somehow get a better wellness plan for me and my life and I have to do whatever it takes, I need to take my power back! I suppose people don't see the effect pain has on me.

Even yesterday, when I proudly declared I don't worry about money, a little later in our chat my friend did ask about my plans for work. 'Out of sight, out of mind,' she said. It's not the first time that has been said to me recently by well-meaning friends. Don't they realise that I had no other option? It wasn't an easy decision for me. I felt that pain had won when I handed in my request for leave. I am only on contract for voice-over work, but effectively I am saying I am not available for my weekly TV slot or to shoot any TV programmes or to cover studio work. I am now OFF.

I feel I had no other option and, as I sit here, I know it was the right thing to do. Andrea, feel proud, confident that from your decision to put your wellness first only good will come!

I am happy with my decision. I will be my own light at the end of my pain tunnel. While I am not pain free yet, I feel for the first time that I will begin a pain management programme, tailor-made for me by myself. Ultimately I feel I will have success with this journey. I have tried other pain management systems; now it's time to trust in me and in my own wisdom. I think the first step for me is to be kind to myself, to focus on the positives and trust in the process. It is good to acknowledge my feelings, accept my feelings; things can only be changed if we recognise we need to change.

Today I embrace change. Blessings & abundance for 2014.

A x

18

New York, New Doctor, New Hope?

Cutting back on my medications in January meant that my head was a bit scattered: partly from the effects of withdrawal, partly because of the additional pain that inevitably followed reducing the meds. I felt really surprised that so many niggling pains returned – my upper back, neck and arms seemed to be a lot worse – and I was really struggling from day to day. I was dreading the long flight to New York, but the thought of finally getting some positive news about my health kept me focused. I was feeling hopeful that whatever Chiari malformation meant for me or my life, I would be able to manage it.

When we arrived in New York we touched base with the institute and they confirmed the appointment, which was in a couple of days. So while David had his meetings, Mum, Brooke and I would take walks in Central Park. The city was covered in a blanket of snow and it was absolutely freezing, but lovely at the same time. My mind was so distracted by the looming appointment that I didn't even want to go shopping in New York during the January sales! The day of the appointment couldn't come quickly enough.

Finally the morning arrived and we were up and out early. It was quite a distance from Manhattan so we travelled in a taxi, which seemed to take for ever. David and I were very quiet during the journey, both just clasping each other's hand, wondering what the doctor would say. I was more than a little fearful, I have to confess.

We got some good news when we arrived; the doctor I had read about would be taking the consultation, which was a very positive start. I looked around at everyone in the waiting area, thinking 'Do they have Chiari?' Some people looked perfectly healthy, some had obvious signs of paralysis, and some needed assistance with mobility. My mind was racing with questions. How can I live pain free? Should I come off these tablets?

Before we saw the doctor I had an in-depth consultation and physical exam with one of the nursing team. Then it was time to meet him, and he immediately put us at our ease, telling us that he had developed a passion for treating Chiari malformation and syringomyelia, and that is what he did every day, so he certainly was the expert I was hoping to meet. He explained that Chiari malformation 1 is a congenital disorder, a defect allowing cerebellar tonsils to herniate (protrude) through the base of the skull. Ten to fifteen years ago it was considered a rare disorder, but advances in MRI scanning and imaging have led to more, and earlier, diagnoses. Today it affects more than two million Americans. He explained that Chiari is widely misunderstood and that there is still limited clinical knowledge about the disorder. He and his team dealt with it every day, and in his experience the clinical presentation of the malformation was so diverse and so complex that very often patients might be seen as hypochondriacs, because their symptoms seem to have an unknown origin. Very often his patients arrived with no diagnosis, so most of them were self-referred, having heard about the institute through word of mouth or their own research into Chiari malformation.

I was a little overwhelmed, and he could probably sense that. He discussed my scan and confirmed it was a Chiari 1. In more easy to understand language he explained, 'Your Chiari malformation is like a car pile-up on a highway. If you can imagine seven lanes in the highway and imagine three of the lanes are involved in a crash, this will allow some lanes to operate normally while others are slower. Your cerebrospinal fluid is only able to flow in four of the seven lanes, and this creates a high-pressure system which can cause many symptoms.' There was a lot to take in, and in hindsight I wish I had recorded it on my phone.

Most of all I was interested in how the pain might be reduced. We went through my symptoms and he confirmed that many were caused by Chiari, even little things such as a mild difficulty swallowing sometimes, which I had previously attributed to tablets and dry mouth. The pins and needles in my hands, sometimes legs, and the inner ear problems I had had since childhood could also be because of the Chiari. I told the doctor about the increased pain in my middle back, neck and shoulder area and he said he had seen this before in Chiari patients. He explained that because Chiari involves the nervous system, symptoms can be numerous and varied.

I felt validated, understood and taken seriously. Maybe all my mysterious pain could be related to this? I didn't feel afraid to reveal all the areas causing me pain or discomfort. Then, feeling hopeful, I asked him about treatment. Was there a cure, a tablet or a procedure to fix this?

He told me that there is no cure yet, but surgery can be an option for Chiari in some cases. 'With surgical treatment the aim is decompression – by removing brain tissue in the opening of the skull, you open the bone at the back of the head to allow the spinal fluid to flow freely. As with any surgery, the chance of success depends on the individual case. Success can mean different things to different people; reduction in pain is success to one person but not to another, who wants to be completely symptom free.' If my symptoms were interfering with quality of life, getting worse, or if the nervous system was being impaired, I could look further into the surgery. But in the meantime there was some medication I could take that would relieve the symptoms.

So we discussed medication. I told him about all the medication I was currently taking and about the particular medication I was hoping to come off. While we were in New York I had tried to reduce it further, against Dr Bleakley's orders, and not as we had planned to do it. I explained this to him, but he advised that I go back on it and wean myself off it more slowly, just as Dr Bleakley had advised. He said that stopping the medication too quickly could make you go 'doolally' and agreed that it would be wise to come off it slowly. He confirmed that one tablet I was on can cause weight gain and make you feel a little spaced out. As for the muscle relaxants, he said that, taken long term, they can affect other muscles. So we had a very interesting chat about medication and he felt I was getting the best advice from my GP, Dr Murphy and the pain management team. I felt empowered, and it made me more determined to stick to my plan to reduce the medication.

David then asked the doctor what the natural progression of Chiari was. He explained that it varies from person to person and is still not well understood, but it can lead to paralysis.

Then I asked, 'What are the odds I would be symptom-free following surgery? And what are the odds I would get worse?'

'The best thing to do is wait and watch. Currently you're mobile, healthy, coping well, managing pain well and keeping positive, so I wouldn't recommend surgery – it would be the last resort. Send me a scan every year to document the progress of the Chiari, keep a diary and monitor your symptoms. Limit activities that might make it worse, or that would leave you open to making it worse. Bungee jumping is out!' He explained that little things like sneezing, blowing my nose and other normal tasks like carrying heavy items could make the head pain worse, so I should be aware of those little actions. He congratulated me on my coping strategies and encouraged me to continue to embrace my own wellness – 'That's the most important thing.' Now that I had had an appointment with him, I was free to email him, ask questions, send on scans. 'I might not get back to you straight away,' he said, 'but I will respond.'

I am very thankful to have met him. He understood my pain and gave me good advice about medication. The whole event really changed something in me. Firstly, I felt he joined a lot of the dots together in my medical history. If I was born with Chiari this could be the underlying cause of all the pain from childhood until now, and would explain why the lumbar punctures had such a serious effect on my body and the reason for the weakness in my upper body. He was so knowledgeable and reassuring about the condition that it took away some of my fear about having this rare malformation. I felt I was in safe hands should I need to explore surgery in the future.

Secondly, after that meeting I started to look to my brain as being the source of my problem and I began to question whether my pain was all in my brain. This was an area I would explore in great detail over the coming months.

Finally, he made me feel really good about how I was managing my situation. Despite everything I had to deal with, I was coping well in his eyes. He spoke briefly about how life-limiting this condition can be, but he congratulated me on my determination to keep going despite the pain, and supported my multidisciplinary wellness plan. I took great positivity from the meeting – I was doing well. I needed to believe in myself more and trust that I could do even better over time, but it wasn't going to be easy.

Pain-*free* Life

February 2014

Pain is a lonely, isolating place to be.

As I took my gentle morning walk in the rain, enjoying the quietness of nature, enjoying my constant companion Dash pottering away, following scents, I had a sad feeling which seemed to just overwhelm me. Living in pain is a lonely life.

Sometimes I really feel so alone with my feelings of pain, it's really hard to ever explain to someone what it feels like. It has been so hard coming off some of my medication again. I did it with the support and guidance of Penny, but it has been so hard. I know it was the right thing to do for me. Medication has its role in the daily management of pain, but personally, I don't like taking it. I spoke to Penny about it and she asked why I wanted to reduce the medication. I gave the usual reasons: it is making me feel foggy, in a haze, removed from what's going on in my body and so on. Plus I want the option of getting pregnant again. We made a plan to wean me off the one tablet that I was very unhappy with. We agreed it would be good to do it now, during my three months off work. I want to do my own home detox plan. I am calling it my 'soul & healing diet'. To be honest a 'diet' seemed like a good way of looking at it, it seemed perfect – after Christmas we are bombarded with 'New Year New You' diet plans and maybe subliminally that affected me. But I did have to eliminate some things; like any 'diet', certain things are not good for you, certainly not healthy. So I had to change my life and introduce good systems and practices into it.

Like any diet I have fallen off the wagon, didn't do my daily affirmations, relaxations, daily walking, writing down my feelings throughout the journey, sticking to my wellness plan, pacing – all those things I agreed with myself at the start of the year I would do without fail. But instead of blaming it on the pain, which I had been doing, I took responsibility, and looking back, that's been one of my biggest lessons in recent weeks. I have the power to change, it's my relationship with 'me, myself, I' that is the key to unlocking this pain cycle.

This time when I reduced the medication I tackled my feelings of depression head on. I could recognise those dark thoughts when they came back this time. Weaning myself off the medication is very scary. For the first week I had a constant feeling of near terror, the horrible dark feeling was back, but I knew if I worked through it, actually allowing those feelings to be, and to recognise them, name them and say 'they are here now', that they would pass.

Another big lesson I have learned over the past month of not being in work and making my health my job daily, is that at the start of January it would have been easy to get wrapped up in a new project. I can still remember when I got the call from Mags asking if I would like to take on a project and I was a little seduced by the prospect of a new challenge, and the financial reward too was all very tempting, but now, a month later, I am feeling so proud I didn't take the job. It would have been another way of side-tracking myself from my main goals this year, another distraction.

So, for the first time ever, I said no to work and yes to myself. My goal was to make my own wellness a full-time job. This is my body, I needed to start taking ownership, taking responsibility for what is happening on the inside. I can't 'blame' pain all the time. I am so thankful I chose to give myself back the power of my own health. If there is anyone who can help me, then surely that person is me!

To be fair, I have a great support network of medical professionals who have been my rocks along the way. Then others, and Carmel, my life healer, who I believe was heaven-sent to heal and offer guidance and advice. I said at the start of the year I needed to be open to all options, look into anything and everything that can help me become well, be willing to really try to achieve all my health goals.

'Gently' is my new word, not 'pacing' anymore, my word is gentle. I do things in a gentle manner and treat myself gently. But all the while I am feeling a little alone. All this stuff I am doing is internal, it's very much a solitary journey, one I have been taking alone, changing my perception and inner dialogue. I am still trying to remove the word 'pain' from my daily speech. This is an idea that has remained with me since the new year, the idea of leaving behind what I don't want, so I am looking for other ways to describe my pain without mentioning the dreaded 'p' word.

But there is still a deep sadness. When I think of how people in pain are treated, I feel we are let down by society. This is a real problem. That is the tragedy I feel with chronic pain, being doubted all the time, constantly having to justify it. Some people, and I include myself, occasionally feel the need to hold their neck or back a certain way, like a physical cue to show the world they are actually in pain.

Having a pain-free life should be part of every human being's basic human rights and I pray for a day when it will be and I hope that pain will be treated with the same urgency as any other serious illness. But until that day I am making it my mission to keep myself well. It is a lonely journey, it is all-consuming right now, but if I can get a really good programme that fits my life and if I can live gently and in balance, my life will be so much more enriched and that's what I am hoping for.

19

Looking for Alternatives

During the months that followed I spent a lot of time thinking about what caused my pain. Was it really the Chiari? Was my pain gate damaged? Was how my mind perceived pain broken? There was such a mismatch in my mind – yes, I felt pain in my body, but mentally I felt strongly there was nothing wrong with me and I would somehow be able to unlock something deep inside my mind that could stop the pain. I wanted to be healed and I didn't want the cure to be in tablet form.

In my daily journal I found myself going over and over different questions. Would scientists one day be able to find out how pain signals are measured in the brain? Is there a connection between pain and our emotions? How do I know that the pain will not have a long-term effect on my brain? Is there any research on people who live in pain every day – will they die early? If all the pain I feel is stemming from and created in the brain, could we retrain our brains not to feel the pain? Why is the pain system damaged? Why is my pain system constantly firing pain to certain areas? What is wrong with my central nervous system?

I really couldn't believe there isn't a cure, or some explanation for why so many people around the world suffer the torture of chronic pain. Having met so many people in person through the hospital and on our private pain forum, I don't know any who are mad – we can't all be imagining it. Most of us have, or at one time had, successful careers, oftentimes spending years honing a craft, working hard to reach a high level in our career paths, only to find that for no reason, or because of an injury that should have healed, we are left with constant, chronic pain.

It would be so easy to allow pain to make your life a constant living nightmare. So I had to be proactive to stay positive. I trawled the Internet, scoured libraries and watched documentaries about healing yourself. Could it be that easy? I looked to Florence Scovel Shinn and Louise L. Hay, I said affirmations over and over again: 'My body now restores itself to its natural state of full health.' I said this positive health statement in the car, walking the dog, making the dinner, over and over in the morning and at night just before going to sleep. I also got a huge sheet of paper and rolled it out to fit from floor to ceiling on my full-length mirror in the bedroom, and with a big black marker I wrote out my affirmations for health and I looked at them while saying them in the mirror over and over again.

Did it work?

Well, it didn't not work!

Yes, I still had pain, but I seemed to be coping better. I had been in such a dark place, but the constant struggle of pushing myself through the pain was certainly gone. At the time everything I was doing was helping.

In order to function day to day and to manage the pain while reducing the medication, I needed to do many things to help control it and to help me deal with life. I focused on the weekly routine things, the daily things, and sometimes the hourly things to stay positive, rather than focusing on the constant pain. I explain this in full in my wellness plan in the second part of this book.

During that time I was exploring many different alternative treatment and healers, and the ones I still use or still see now are the ones that worked for me. I spent a lot of time, money and energy trying everything anyone suggested. As most people living with chronic pain will confirm, everything is worth exploring.

Around this time I interviewed Katie Jane Goldin on my radio show on Sunshine 106.8 about her late father, the famous hypnotist Paul Goldin. We spoke at length about the power of the mind and her late father's own incredible story. After the interview we chatted at length, and she very kindly suggested that I come to the clinic for a session. I had tried hypnosis videos online and had read about how it had been successful in treating many medical conditions. Some patients even use hypnosis for pain management during surgery, and people had even had complicated dental work done under hypnosis.

I was intrigued. If all the pain I feel is stemming from and being created in the brain, could I retrain my brain not to feel the pain? I called the clinic and spoke to Helen Goldin, Paul's widow, who now runs the clinic with Katie Jane. She was very easy to talk to, and I opened up to her about my wellness journey. She seemed to have a great understanding of and empathy for patients with chronic pain. So I was very excited about the appointment the following week.

March 2014

Chronic pain: what's the alternative?

I have been thinking a lot recently about the very many different things I have done over the past vast number of years to try to stop the pain.

This morning I asked my trusted pain friends on my private Facebook chronic pain group, 'Has anyone heard about using turmeric for pain?' I got some wonderful responses so as I headed out to the shop to buy copious amounts of the healing spice, I was feeling very excited and a little hopeful. I was planning a big cooking afternoon so I could add the fragrant spice to every meal imaginable, as I had read on the web that it was good for inflammation – granted, it was an animal website I was on, but if it is good for joint pain I would give it a go. As I drove to the shop I was in a trance.

I was contemplating rubbing it all over my body, then I was thinking I would need a few jars of the stuff, so as my mind wandered a bit, I remembered previous experiences of using it in cooking, the lovely stain it leaves on everything it touches … so I started to rethink the idea of rubbing it all over my body. But that got me thinking of how often I have tried random things or gone to so many people hoping to get some relief for my pain.

If David came home to see me sitting in the bath covered in sweet-smelling turmeric he would probably think I was mad. But these are the mad things you find yourself googling – and sometimes doing – to get rid of the pain. So tomorrow, for example, I plan to have a consultation at a hypnosis clinic to see if they can address my chronic pain through hypnosis. I have been promised, with 100 per cent certainty, they can and will help. So tomorrow I will be face to face, yet again, with a stranger asking questions about my life, my pain, what I have tried, what I haven't tried, how I feel, how does it affect my life. How? When? Where?

And they will ask that question, the one I don't really have an answer for but that I'd really like to have: Why?

So because I don't have the 'why', and I haven't cracked how to get rid of it completely, I will have to tell a stranger tomorrow morning all about me and my pain. Nonetheless I am hopeful.

Mind over matter?

I believe in the power of the mind. I suppose that's why I can't get my head around the fact that I still have pain. Why can't I just use the power of positive thinking to overcome it?

Hand in hand with my first hypnosis session tomorrow I am going to see a lady who I regularly visit, we can call her my alternative 'healer'. I have been seeing Carmel now for a while. She was recommended to me by various people so I decided to give it a try and, honestly, I do feel she has healing powers, as I feel many people who walk the earth do.

So tomorrow, when I am with my healer Carmel, I will be on the bed after our chat, where I will smell an oil, try to close my eyes and relax, then get Reiki and kinesiology healing, listen to affirmations, say my name and repeat, 'I am at base clean and good', 'My future is safe and secure', 'I am jumping with joy', then loud bells will chime and we will do a close down. This is all part of how I deal with my pain, this is part of Andrea's programme for managing her pain.

And feck what people think, because it all really helps me.

So for anybody who thinks we are mad, or imagining the pain or think it's all in our head, seriously, do you think I want to be covered in turmeric? To tell a stranger my life story so I can play a recording at night to be hypnotised? To travel all around the country to see alternative healers? And the thing is, sometimes desperate people like me who are dealing with chronic pain are easily taken advantage of. I promise you, over the years I have spent too much money looking for a cure, whether it was to be found at the end of a bottle, on top of a treatment table, in a gym, by swallowing supplements, going to a healer, a physio, a doctor or with a past life regression therapist … Honestly.

I am little ashamed of some of the crazy, wacky things I have done. As I type, I am laughing out loud at the memory of one particular occasion. I drove out of the city to a remote place down the country. With some difficulty I managed to find the isolated house. At the end of a country lane I parked the car and was greeted by a fairly solid man. He looked a bit menacing. Directed by his hand gestures I followed him past his house, down the back of the garden, into a darker, almost wooded area and into a wooden shed! After a chat, telling yet another stranger about my life and all about my pain, he said that I had a curse on me. That's when it got very weird. I stood up, faced the wall with an image of an ascended master! As requested, I spread my arms and legs and the man, behind me, started chanting and blowing on me. I could hear him clapping every so often too. Trust me, it wasn't relaxing, all I could think of was that I had left my phone in the car and that no one knew I was here, not even David. Suddenly panic took over. I could be killed and no one would know where to start to find me! Thankfully, it was over quickly and I ran out of the place. I promised myself not to go to any 'healers' again. Clearly I didn't keep that promise because hope wins out sometimes!

I think it all helps. If it makes me better equipped to deal with the day-to-day grind of pain, then it will be a good day. I shall report back!

My first visit to the clinic was on a crisp sunny spring morning; there were lovely flowers in bloom outside and I thought that maybe this was a new beginning for me, the start of something really good. A lovely lady greeted me with a warm welcome and took me into a room to fill out some forms. Before each session you write down a list of goals, of what you hope to achieve from the hypnosis. My goals were simple and clear – pain reduction, better sleep. I then went into another room with a lovely big cosy chair and met my therapist, Mary. We had a long chat about me, my reasons for being there and what the therapy involved. She explained that hypnosis is an excellent focusing mechanism for patients with pain. It all sounded too good to be true.

So what is hypnosis? It's probably not what you think. Stage hypnosis, which we are all familiar with, and the practical application of hypnosis are very different. Hypnosis is a relaxed state of attentive concentration. Hypnosis is *not* sleep. When you are in hypnosis you are awake and alert, but you feel deeply and pleasantly relaxed. And when you are deeply relaxed, you cannot feel uncomfortable.

Mary explained that I would be guided to focus away from discomfort or pain and to re-focus on comfort and pleasant sensations. My first therapist-led hypnosis session, to my surprise, was very relaxing and a really wonderful experience. I was surprised how long it was – almost thirty minutes – but it felt as though just ten minutes had passed. Mary explained that time distortion is often common during deep relaxation.

I arranged to come back at the same time the following week and was sent home with a hypnosis CD, which I was told I should listen to every morning before getting out of bed and every evening before I went to sleep. I often found I was listening to it during the day too. I didn't feel a massive decrease in pain, but I did enjoy the sense of deep relaxation.

For my second session I had to fill in the form again, saying what I wanted to achieve and how I had felt since the last session. I felt more positive and that the CD was helping with my sleep patterns. If I did experience broken sleep, instead of lying awake thinking of the pain and how I was awake yet again, I listened to the CD and found it easier to drift back to sleep or into a pleasant state of deep relaxation.

I had ten more sessions with Mary and during that time we worked through many areas in my life, from weight loss to confidence and lots of pain-related issues. One of the issues that we tackled I hadn't ever discussed or in truth really acknowledged to myself. Often I would unconsciously pick at the skin around my neck or jawline, usually when I was feeling pain in my neck or shoulders, and sometimes I would scratch until I bled. I hadn't really looked at why I did this, but it was because of the pain – it was almost a distraction tactic. That was the perfect thing to work on with Mary, and she gave me some diversions to think of when I felt my hand lifting to my face. I was so happy that I could work through issues in hypnosis with such success.

I really feel that my sessions with such a skilled therapist and my determination to do what I was told and actually make the commitment to listen as directed to the hypnosis CDs made a big difference. It was a big part of my home pain management routine during those crucial months that followed.

The success of those sessions led me to ask myself, is pain subjective? Does the answer lie deep in our minds? Could it be so simple that listening to the continuous reinforcement of positive messages on a hypnosis CD could penetrate our subconscious minds, so that, maybe, we could be cured of pain? I wanted to delve into the whole notion of mind over matter.

20

Returning to Work

At the beginning of April I returned to work, but I was different. Two major changes unfolded that led to a massive breakthrough for me, both mentally and physically. The first change was in work. The second was my decision to change the way I thought about and referred to my pain.

When I left work in January a newspaper article revealed that I had taken time off to have more family time and to take care of my chronic pain, so on my return many people believed I was cured. As I learned, being upbeat and happy doesn't really match up with someone who has chronic pain. The picture that had accompanied the piece I wrote for *Woman's Way* was a smiling photo of me with a dog, and someone later said to me that the picture didn't really 'do anything' for chronic pain, that it didn't really convey what being in chronic pain meant or felt like. I struggled with this concept for a while – should I be depressed or sad to reflect the pain I feel?

As a society we are afraid of pain – it means that something is wrong and we are taught that it is a consequence of something else. Find the source or cause of the pain, then treat it, and the pain will go. Generally when people who are not used to chronic pain experience pain they are not happy – they take time off work, moan and groan (understandably so), and it is clear to everyone that they are in pain. I felt that because I was jolly and positive some people didn't see my pain as real, or serious.

It can be hard to stay positive about the fact that this pain really defies explanation. I find myself explaining and re-explaining it to new people as they come into my life; explaining that although I am in and out of hospital, I'm not really getting any better; that I don't even know if I *will* get better. And when their questions stop, I find I start questioning myself. It makes me think about just how different I feel from others and really how most people, even my good friends and family, have no concept of how I (and many others like me) suffer with pain daily. It is an invisible illness, so sufferers can choose to try to hide it or to talk to people about it. If you do try to talk about it, you often find that as much as people might think they understand, like anything in life, you really don't know what it is like until you live it every day.

After three months of focusing on my complete wellness I felt a lot better, but I realised that this wasn't going to be a quick fix. In general I had a low level of pain every day, but sometimes it could be more intense – a feeling like muscle spasms, quite sharp, almost like a burning or gnawing. But I was having these pain flare-ups less and less, and I felt really happy that I was having more good days than bad. While I was off work I managed my pain really well – when I have a flare-up I generally feel fatigued and for the first time I was able to rest when this happened. Instead of becoming so exhausted that I would crash and burn, as I had so many times in the past, I took time out to actively rest. I would listen to my hypnosis CD to recoup my energy or take a guided meditation. I definitely felt a lot better overall, and it seemed that sticking to my own rigid pain management at home was actually making a difference.

Not surprisingly, as the end of my leave approached I was feeling a little nervous. I worried that all my good routines might be difficult to maintain alongside the demands of work. However, when the day came to go back to work I was feeling very upbeat, positive and quietly hopeful that I would be able to juggle it all.

I enjoyed my work, so it was nice to be back in the familiar busy environment of a TV station. Very little had changed and I easily slipped back into the flow of work again. It was a long first day, as I was catching up with colleagues, and many people thought I was 'looking great' after my three-month sabbatical. In the past I felt as though I had become an expert at disguising my pain at work – it was how I coped – but looks can be deceiving. Hiding behind my make-up and my smile, I was still in pain.

On that first day back many people asked me, 'Is your back better?' How should I answer? Normally I would have lied and said, 'I'm grand.' This time I found myself thinking about my new pain management plan. I knew I would need to factor changes into my working day to allow me to continue with my new way of managing my pain, so I asked myself if I should be more honest about that pain. I would need support from colleagues, so should I explain that yes, my back hurts, but so do my arms, hands, legs, feet, sometimes my head and even my eyes? The list could go on and on, and the symptoms change in severity daily because chronic pain is very complex. To answer their question honestly, should I say, 'My back isn't better, neither is my damaged pain system, and there is still no cure for my rare disorder, Chiari malformation'? I hadn't even told anyone about that yet! On that first day I decided it would be too exhausting trying to explain to people about my pain, so generally I told people I was feeling good. But as the days went on, deciding what to tell people kept me awake at night.

A week later I was reflecting on my first week back at work while I took my morning walk. I hadn't slept well, as my pain level was really up. Part of the problem was that my work space wasn't ideal. I shared a 'hot desk' with a number of others. Any attempt to keep the seat, screen or keyboard in a certain way for my physical comfort wasn't an option, as others might move chairs around; in fact, my back support was here today and gone the next. Oftentimes someone was waiting to use the computer or trying to get into the voice-over booth. This meant that instead of taking breaks and pacing, in that first week I was gritting my teeth and working through really bad pain, afraid that if I moved away I would lose my 'slot'. In fact some new systems had been put in place which meant we had more administrative scheduling work to accompany our voice-overs. I was spending less time doing voice-overs in the studio and more time entering data, which wasn't helping my arm pain.

I felt very strongly that I needed to continue on my journey to discover more about myself and about my pain; I needed to explore more ways to heal from within. I knew I had made a mental shift about the pain, and I felt that if I could just research it a bit more and try additional ways to control the pain I would reap the benefits.

I was deep in my own little world as I walked into the dog park. I wasn't saying 'Good morning' to anyone that day. I was trying to be invisible, let Dash have a run around and avoid any contact with anyone. As the dogs played I found myself reluctantly joining a group and there was a little bit of polite morning chat. Then one of the women said, 'I know you.' I prayed inwardly, 'Please don't talk to me this morning, I'm really not feeling able to chat.' With the increased pain I didn't feel I could even be polite, but what she said next really surprised me. She told me she had read my article on chronic pain in *Woman's Way* magazine and it had had a hugely positive effect on her life. She went on to thank me for writing it and for sharing my story. She told me that this was her first day out of her house in over two weeks. I didn't say anything, but my face probably spoke volumes. She asked me, 'How do you do it?' and I replied, 'Today, with great difficulty, but you just need to keep going.' I explained that in recent months it had been easier as I had been off work and didn't have massive demands on me, but I had recently returned to work and today wasn't a good day.

She became visibly upset when she told me she hadn't worked for a long time and felt very isolated. She didn't think her family or friends truly believed her symptoms. I totally understood, but I couldn't talk to her as long as I wanted to. My head felt like a ton weight grinding down on my shoulders and I almost couldn't talk, so I wished her well and left the park.

As I continued walking I was so annoyed at myself; I was angry that my body was in pain this morning. I would normally want to talk to a fellow sufferer, say some encouraging words, but today I just felt like I wanted to go into a dark room, close the door on the world and be in bed. I desperately hated feeling this way. I started to cry silently, shedding tears of sadness that pain had made me like this. In my head I was screaming, 'I am not like that.' I am a caring, sociable and chatty person, but that morning the pain had won. Then, as I walked, unable to even wipe my tears away, I was reminded why I first wrote the article – acceptance! I had a sudden moment of complete clarity: would I once more be sugar-coating the pain at work if I wasn't honest about it and how it affected me daily?

It was clear to me that my current situation wasn't working, I couldn't possibly continue on in work as if I was 'normal', living without pain. My mind raced and I recalled a conversation I had had with a colleague, who had asked if I would consider redundancy. I must admit it wasn't the 'Welcome back' I was hoping for, but I suddenly thought that maybe it was worth exploring. Should I apply to leave permanently? Had pain made me redundant? More tears fell and it started to rain.

Pain-*free* Life

Gratitude diary

April 2014

Thank you for the wonderful team of doctors and nurses in Vincent's, I am so lucky to have such support and understanding from Dr Murphy, and of course a great GP. Penny has been brilliant; I don't think I could have got through recent months without her. I am so grateful for the support of my 'pain friends' on Facebook. I have connected with some lovely people all over the country and although I haven't met them I know they understand and are always there to listen to my ranting without judgement, which I appreciate so much. Thank you for friendship. I am so blessed with my wonderful patient, caring husband. Thank you most sincerely for Brooke. I feel very lucky that I have believed in myself in recent months and I have trusted my inner guidance about my wellness. I have gratitude tonight for every cell in my body and my vibrant health. Bless my family, friends, doctors, nurses and everyone who has helped me along the way, especially my earth angel Dash. Archangel Michael, continue to watch over me and give me strength and a positive outlook to count my blessings always. Angel Daniel, watch over my marriage. A x

21

Embracing Change

Once again I was thinking of leaving a job that I really enjoyed. I struggled with my decision to apply for redundancy. David, as always, was so supportive; he could see the positive changes in me physically and mentally, and he encouraged me to continue on my journey of wellness. We even talked about the possibility of studying hypnosis or looking at other options for work that wouldn't involve as much computer work. We agreed that I could explore more TV work in due course but, ultimately, he said, 'Your health is your wealth, so if you feel this will help you manage your pain I will support you. But only you can make the decision.'

He was right. It was my decision and I had to do it for the right reasons. Of course, being at home and spending time with Brooke would be amazing, but was it the pain that was making me leave or did I just want to be at home with Brooke – or both? I began to torture myself and my inner self talk became very negative. 'Is my pain bad enough for me to give up work? Why isn't there a test that can measure the severity of the pain a person feels? If only I could compare and contrast my pain to someone else's pain, would others who experience this pain work through it?' This was a massive hurdle to get my mind over. I felt that in some ways I was constantly battling the misconceptions others had about my invisible pain. How I looked physically was a far cry from how I was actually feeling, but my pain was something I hid very well and now it seemed to be taking control of my life once again.

With a heavy heart, at the end of April 2014 I decided to apply for redundancy. I found myself sitting in the HR office of TV3 explaining my reasons. We discussed my chronic pain and my recent diagnosis of Chiari malformation and, naturally, there were questions. I explained that my symptoms would not be exactly the same as another person's, but the most dominant symptom, and the one we all share, is body pain. I think it was a big surprise for me to be as candid as I was. I was considered a very positive person in TV3: always sending angel cards to people and generally laughing and joking. Opening up about my constant battle with pain was a shock to many. I remember explaining that just getting up and looking presentable every day took a lot of energy, and lots of caffeine too. Sometimes it might take me two hours to get out of the house because I had to stop and rest after washing my hair or putting on eye make-up. These simple tasks caused such an increase in arm, neck and shoulder pain that each became a massive chore.

So it was done. I applied for redundancy and it was agreed. I was asked if I could give twelve weeks' notice, to allow time to find and train a replacement. This was a lot longer than I had expected, but I agreed. I knew then that to maintain the best possible balance over the weeks ahead I would need to stick rigidly to my plan, increase my relaxation and stretches, and try to explore additional ways to stay on top of the pain.

My research into wellness took me to many different websites and I read various books on healing. I delved into the placebo effect, read a study on the effects of healers on physiological outcomes in patients, the healing powers of prayer and the science behind meditation, which proves that it has an effect on well-being and can reduce pain – real-life miracles. I cast my net far and wide and became engrossed in collecting everything and anything that could work on pain. That's when I had a major breakthrough.

I had been listening to guided hypnoses and meditations for pain for many months and I felt that some of the scripts could be better. Pain is a lot more sophisticated than the people who developed these realised; probably because they don't fully understand the experience of chronic pain. I often feel that it is far more complex than even the medical profession understand. In a moment of inspiration I began to write a script that would be tailor-made for my pain and my own daily experience of it. At TV3 I wrote scripts for continuity every day, I've scripted TV shows, I script my radio talk show every week, so it is something that comes easily to me. There was one major change, however: I decided I didn't want to refer to my pain any more. I was taking control and pain wasn't going to be centre stage in my script. In fact, I wrote, 'You do not have pain, you do not want chronic pain, Andrea, and you are not accepting the experience of pain any more.' Instead I referred to 'sensations'; my pain was merely a 'sensation' and I could control these in my body.

At the time I didn't realise what a profound effect this change would have on me, but it was a game changer. I recorded a twenty-five-minute script on my iPhone. Surprisingly, I did it in one take – it was perfect. For many, reading twenty-five minutes of a script might be a daunting task, but I was an experienced voice-over artist. I wondered why I hadn't thought of it sooner!

But would it work?

That night, instead of my usual night-time hypnosis, I listened to my recording. At the start it was a little strange, but hearing myself repeat all the positive suggestions became empowering. I was much more receptive to the ideas for healing when I heard them in my own voice. Plus I understood pain, so the language felt real: subconsciously that had to have a deeper healing effect in the hypnosis!

Was it even proper hypnosis? Probably not, but guess what, it worked. I fell asleep while listening to it. When uncomfortable 'sensations' woke me I listened again and, while I didn't fall asleep, I felt very relaxed and positive. Was I on to something? The next day I listened to it again morning and night, in fact I followed the same pattern and routine as if it were a new recording I had been given by the Paul Goldin Clinic. I tried to listen at least three times a day. To reinforce the idea of not having pain I started to write out healing affirmations, removing the word 'pain' and saying that I would be 'sensation free'.

The repetition seemed to have an effect. I noticed that when I was having my usual inner dialogue about the day and how I was feeling I would refer to my pain as 'sensations' – there was no mention of pain. Could changing my inner narrative have a long-term effect on my pain? Could the language I used for my pain actually be part of the problem? The word 'pain' has such negative connotations, for me it felt much easier to reject the word and replace it with 'sensations', or 'pressure' or 'heaviness'.

So I was pain free in my mind. I continued to listen to my own hypnosis and made a decision to study it formally. I asked Helen Goldin who she would consider a good teacher, given that her late husband had been Ireland's leading hypnotherapist and had had a huge interest in its application in medicine. She told me about a wonderful teacher called Niamh Flynn, from the Galway Clinic, who works as a trainer for the National Guild of Hypnotists, the largest and oldest hypnotherapy membership organisation in the world. I was really excited that I was going to formally explore the power of the mind. As I had committed to working until August I booked a place on a course in September.

Maybe now I could find a way of decreasing and managing the elusive pain that had become the bane of my everyday existence. I could never quite grasp the pathology underlying my pain: was it spinal stenosis, as diagnosed in London; facet degeneration; prolapsed discs; or Chiari malformation? The pain I experienced never seemed to match the possible cause – it defied logic. For now, though, I created more of my own guided affirmations and relaxations and truly changed my language of pain. This really helped me get through those last weeks in work.

Although I was exploring alternative therapies, I wasn't ignoring traditional medicine. In August I had my appointment at the Poynton Spine Care Institute in the Mater Hospital in Dublin to get advice on surgical options from neurosurgeon Ashley Poynton. When the morning arrived for the appointment I was feeling very positive, in a hopeful frame of mind after my healing hypnosis and positive affirmations. Mr Poynton's offices aren't located in the hospital itself, so I had to find my way from the parking lot in the rain. My sense of direction failed me: I was lost and stressed and began to run. My gentle approach went out the window and, needless to say, my sensations increased and I reached for my trusted pain meds. In a way it was a good thing because it reminded me how quickly things can change and how wonderful life would be without pain. Maybe surgery could be a good option.

When I finally got to my appointment we had a very in-depth meeting and assessment; Mr Poynton noticed some muscle wastage in my arms and wrist, which surprised me, as I didn't understand how he could see it so clearly. He felt I would be a good candidate for cervical neck surgery: 'We could remove discs and build them back up, which would alleviate the pain, but like everything, there is no guarantee.' He felt that the problems could be from the discs, not the Chiari. He had treated Chiari before and had excellent knowledge of the malformation, which was reassuring. He explained that the surgery would be via my throat, which was worrying as I used my voice box for a living, and that could be affected long term, but again I was assured that though damage can happen, it is rare. Overall I felt he was very honest and upfront about everything. I explained my pain management system and how well I felt I was coping. He said, 'Let's just wait and watch,' much like the doctor I had seen in the States. He suggested I send him an updated scan in a year and we could schedule another meeting to see if things had degenerated further.

I now felt more invested than ever in my own alternative pain management plan and that I was making great strides with my personal complementary and alternative approach. It worked for me and seemed to strike the right balance. I had always felt that the healthcare system is primarily medication-centred, and I really didn't want to start increasing any medications. I liked my whole-person healing approach to chronic pain, and I was exploring my own model for wellness and living sensation-free! Trusting my own inner wisdom was central to my success, as was the massive shift in how I perceived and spoke about my pain or 'sensations'.

Giving up my job was the catalyst for me to truly explore my healing potential. Far from being superfluous, I was suddenly very much needed in the creation of my new life without pain. I was now, at least in my mind, living pain free.

August 2014

It was a beautiful summer's day today and I am really enjoying all the beautiful colour that seems to be blooming everywhere in nature. My daily walk today really made me think about how far I have come along this wellness journey. In January, much like the winter season, I felt barren, almost devoid of life, everything seemed grey in my world. I felt bleak, like the backdrop of nature that I walked in every day. The weather was cold, the ground was hard, rain was falling, all the plants and trees were bare, some appeared to be dead. In a way there wasn't much sign of life in my world, I was struggling to see any light. My mind felt much like the dead soil filled with weeds – I knew I needed to be patient, replace the negative weeds in my mind and sow new seeds of positivity. It was the genesis of my new way of managing pain. It was all on me, I was following my own inner guidance. At the time I didn't know if the roots of my new ideas would be a strong enough foundation for my wellness. Could I really create my own plan? I felt I was slowly transforming the landscape of my mind, nourishing it with positive thoughts and new patterns for managing my pain daily. As the seasons transformed, so did I, mentally and physically. When spring arrived, I too started to feel energised and encouraged by the little shoots of change I started to see. A new me was beginning to blossom and grow. New ideas were hatching in my mind, the darkness started to turn to light and my days became a little longer too, as I was enjoying a little bit more of my life every day, by confidently taking ownership of my pain. I seemed to have a new awakening and I wanted to explore even more ways of changing my pain. These harvested even more change and I continued to grow and transform.

Finally, today, it sort of dawned on me that I am abloom, much like the flowers, trees and plants and all of nature. There has been a massive transformation in me. Could I have predicted or even imagined how beautiful life could be for me during those dark days in January? Maybe I was searching for a temporary solution, but I know now this is a lifelong relationship that I need to constantly nourish every day. I feel my mind is like the soil in the ground – nothing can grow in an unproductive and negative mind. You have to trust that the little seeds will grow. Even small changes daily can create massive change – it isn't visible at first and in the past I might have given up just before the little seed or sign of change would be manifest.

I have spent recent weeks focusing on being 'sensation free', controlling my sensations, which has been so empowering. But I decided today, as I enjoyed the beauty of my surroundings, this summer I am going to be sensational!

Another mind shift – I can't have any negativity attached to any sensations! I am embracing how wonderful it is to take control of your sensations! Positive and negative. I am going to actively seek out the good sensations. I even stopped to smell a fragrant white wild rose on my wander today. It felt sensational!

My Wellness Plan

22

You are not your Illness or Pain

Making the journey from patient to person takes time; in my case, a lot more time than I had anticipated, and it is a journey I continue daily. It isn't all calm waters; in fact isolation, fear, anger and just dealing with the pain can overwhelm a person who is living with persistent pain, and it can be very difficult to overcome those negative emotions, particularly at the beginning. So in this section of the book I am going to share the practical details of my journey in the hope that it will help others facing a similar situation. I will reveal what has worked for me and share my personal healing tools, because they are the fruits of my success.

In many ways it has been my lifelong battle with chronic pain that brought me to the inner knowledge that I had to approach me and my pain differently. The most significant breakthrough I made in my journey was that I realised the most important person in my team of medical professionals was me. I trusted that I had the answers within me to feel well again and I embarked on a voyage of self-discovery.

After I was diagnosed with Chiari malformation 1, I had to change and make changes. An inner voice was screaming at me, 'Andrea! Wake up! Take action! *You* need to be the change you are looking for.' So at the beginning of 2014 I focused on living the best life possible, blessing my body and working with it to create perfect balance. I started to refer to my pain as 'sensations'.

I was determined to find the key to unlock the cycle of pain I was living in.

I believe you too can do this. Remember, you are still the same loving person that the universe created. Yes, your life is very difficult and you are faced with many obstacles. However, you have now taken control of your life and your pain. You are strong, and with your new daily wellness plan you will develop a positive mindset to help you cope and work through the various phases of your pain. You hold the key to unlocking the pain and opening the door to the rest of your life. Here are some pointers to help you start the process:

1. Accept the experience of chronic pain and find a good team of people to support you.

If you suffer from severe, chronic pain you know how it can utterly disrupt and damage your life and relationships. Contrary to popular belief, all pain is real. This may seem like an obvious statement, but people with chronic pain are sometimes treated as if their pain is either imaginary or exaggerated. In some cases they feel as though they have to prove their chronic pain to their friends, family and doctors. There are also still some in the medical profession who believe that pain is always a manifestation of an underlying injury or disease. So many doctors focus on treating the underlying cause of the pain, with the belief that once the injury or disease is cured the chronic pain will disappear. If no underlying cause can be found for the pain, the patient is told that very few treatments are available or, worse, 'the pain must be in your head'.

If you don't have support from your doctor or GP, it is time to get a new one. It's okay to change doctors! If you feel your doctor is unresponsive, doesn't understand, or you're simply uncomfortable with them, make the change. Try to find a doctor who specialises in your problem. You will find advice about support groups and pain management programmes online, but finding an understanding GP is essential, so when you meet your new doctor, don't hold back on how you feel, especially about your pain level, types of pain, variations in frequency, sensation and how it affects your daily activities. Your doctor can't help you if they don't have the full picture.

2. Educate yourself about your condition.

It is tempting to go online and search everything to do with your pain, but my advice is not to let it consume all your time, and don't get paranoid looking for new symptoms. It is all about balance. A little information is very useful, but try to keep it positive without dwelling on the symptoms. It can also be helpful to keep up to date about what is happening in the world of medical research and the treatment of chronic pain. My advice is to try to keep a level head about things: the Internet is great but you can't get too bogged down with everything you read. I found that information about alternative treatments that might help or alleviate pain made for interesting reading. I remember reading, 'Joy is portable. I choose to bring it with me today,' and that was often my daily mantra in those days of readjustment.

3. Seek support.

Whether it's via online support groups or one-to-one counselling, find support. When I first found out about support groups it was a revelation and it happened quite by chance. I was messaged on Facebook by someone who spotted that I had liked articles about chronic pain, and this Facebook friend (who I didn't know personally) asked me if I would like to join a small private

Facebook group of people who suffered chronic pain. I was sceptical. I didn't even know you could have a private group on Facebook, and I was a little concerned that my comments might be made public, but I had no reason to worry. The support and peace of mind I got from being a member of the group was amazing. Our experiences were so similar. Together we laugh, cry, support and encourage each other and, although I haven't met most of them, I feel we are true friends.

There are many support groups out there, so find one that you feel comfortable in and you will find that your often lonely experiences will resonate with the other members. A gentle word of warning, though; make sure your group is positive and inclusive, as well as supportive. If you don't feel the people share the same values as you, don't be afraid to leave. There is nothing worse than joining a group for support and finding that you are being judged, so if that's the case, look for another group. You can also find out if there are any local meetings or courses that might help.

One of the most satisfying things about doing the in-patient pain management programme was the interaction with other patients who also had chronic pain. When you meet people who totally understand, it can be just an amazing feeling, particularly if you have been isolated.

When I moved on to doing my pain management at home, I felt I needed that support from the online groups – so thank you to all my 'pain pals' (you know who you are) for the many chats, cards, good wishes, advice, laughs and, most of all, acceptance, friendship and support.

4. Keep up daily activity.
Do not isolate yourself. Try to live as normally as you can. It

is sometimes so hard just to get out of bed and some days you might feel like pulling the covers over your head and ignoring the world for a day or two. This is the time when you need to motivate yourself to take action and get up! I try to get out for a walk every day, rain, hail, wind or shine. When you greet your neighbours, don't talk about your illness or pain. For the short time you are out of the house, focus on the positives. You are outside and taking in all that nature has to offer. I have two walks that I do regularly. One takes about twenty minutes and the other about forty minutes. I know the routes well and I don't have to walk up hills. My routine changed when my daughter started a new school; I found a suitable walk close to the new school so I can still get my daily walk in after dropping her off. Plan for change and leave yourself no excuses for not doing your walk every day.

If you can't do the hobbies you once enjoyed, try a new one. Maybe join a local group or library. Look for adjustments or changes you can make to ease yourself back into society. It can be daunting at first, but once you find something that suits you it can add so much enjoyment to your life. Don't become a recluse, despite the fact you may feel lonely at times, and if you're reading this thinking, 'If I do exercise it will cause more pain, I will feel better if I stay in bed' – keep reading!

5. Be aware of your fear avoidance.

I first learned about fear avoidance and its consequences for chronic musculoskeletal pain when I went to my first pain management course. The whole concept makes perfect sense now, but at first it was a revelation to me. I learned how people often allow pain to take over their lives. The pain sufferer will stop or avoid things that they believe will make the pain more severe, so by allowing the fear of additional pain to take over, they stop doing activities like exercise or travelling or driving. Thinking this way will lead to isolation and your world will slowly close in around you. So ask yourself, am I avoiding activities for fear it will make things worse? When you understand that fear avoidance is common in sufferers of chronic pain and must be overcome, chat to your GP about taking up new activities and get their advice. I had to look at my own life and accept that there was a lot of fear – there still is today and I need to check in with my feelings daily to try to keep grounded about the fear.

6. Managing your pain is all about pacing and spacing activities.
Pacing is a technique that you can use to gradually increase your level of activity. Realise that, while you may feel energised and well one day, instead of overdoing it with a busy schedule, you should try to pace yourself. Do little bits, rather than doing too much and then crashing and burning later on. Understanding these patterns in chronic pain really helped me. When I feel a reduction in the daily pain I have so much energy, my mood is positive and I think I can take on the world, so in the past I would try to pack as much into my day as possible. Knowing not to do this has helped me avoid flare-ups of pain.

Flare-ups, dramatic increases in pain levels, are part of chronic pain. Sadly, you just have to accept them. At the beginning, before the pain management course, I would get very worried and anxious about the increase in pain, but now I know it will pass and I try to have a plan of action ready so that I can cope better. My doctor understands my chronic pain and she might prescribe some muscle relaxants. If you are having regular patterns of flare-up, or a yo-yoing cycle of pain, when you seem to be constantly dealing with heightened pain, then a slight reduction for a few days and then a spike of heightened pain again, you need to talk to your doctor about a plan to manage the flare-ups.

Look at your lifestyle too, as many things can add to your pain flare-ups.

7. Understand yourself.

Pain increases in times of stress. While this is true, what causes stress in one person may be of little concern to another. When I experience a spike in my pain I look at my life and see if there is a reason for the flare-up. I will reveal later how I try to evaluate triggers that might cause me extra stress, and explain the tools and techniques I now use daily to stay calm and positive, but I know this is easier said than done. I really feel as though my emotions directly affect my physical well-being. By acknowledging and dealing with your feelings, you can reduce stress and possibly decrease the pain you feel.

8. Help others to understand you.

Other people's understanding of your circumstances is key when you have chronic pain. It is normal to feel angry, helpless, hopeless and alone. It is important, though, to seek help in dealing with these feelings. Tell your spouse, partner or a family member about how you feel. Make sure you have someone to reach out to, someone you can trust and someone with whom you can share your feelings in an honest way. Sometimes, it is difficult for family members to understand that your pain can make you more impatient and that, as the pain intensifies, it can trigger outbursts of anger or anxiety. It is important to talk to your loved ones at this time, just to let them know it's not directed at them personally and that you are doing the very best you can to manage your pain. As I have mentioned, I found online support groups fantastic for both support and sound advice from people who truly understand what you are going through.

9. Be gentle.

Treat yourself as you would a little child who is in pain, or your best friend if they needed you. Remember to be good to yourself. Chronic pain has a serious impact on the quality of life. You can choose to allow your world to be fuelled by pain and negativity, or you can choose to keep your thoughts and emotions positive. How you feel and think today will affect your experience tomorrow. You need to take control of your life in a positive way. Look beyond your pain to the things that are important in your life. Setting small priorities and making small changes every week can help you find a starting point to lead you back into finding balance again in your life and ultimately to a wellness routine that works for you.

10. Develop a strategy for wellness.

Staying focused on the positives in your life and developing daily coping strategies is essential. But we need to move beyond that and focus a little more on becoming well and staying well. In the following chapters I share what I do to help me stay on top of pain and outline the components of my own 'self-management wellness journey'.

23

Your Wellness Inventory

The term 'wellness' is generally used to mean a healthy balance of the mind, body and spirit that results in an overall feeling of well-being. For me, wellness means the opposite of illness and pain. It isn't just about my health, it's about my well-being in all areas of my life. So it is a combination of things, including spiritual wellness, social wellness, mental wellness, emotional wellness, physical wellness and even pain wellness. I want to live my best possible life, to feel in balance and to feel well.

I suppose 'pain wellness' is hard to define – there is no set standard. This chapter is about your perception of wellness. What pain wellness might mean for you may be different from what it means to someone else. For me, having low pain is a good place to be in. I wanted to reduce my pain sensations with the hope of, maybe, living without pain.

In January 2014 I sat in my bedroom going through my life as I would in pre-production for a new show. I was looking into every area of my life hoping to 'produce' it better by asking myself certain questions:

- Are you generally happy? What makes you happy? What would make you happier?

- What would you do if anything were possible? Are you content with life? Is this how you want to live your life? Is your life in balance? What would be your idea of perfect

- balance? Do you live with joy and love? Are you in a healthy, harmonious relationship?

- Are you generally sad? Why do you feel sad? Do you feel trapped? Why do you feel trapped?

- Are you stressed? What adds to your stress? How could you live with less stress in your life?

- Do you live with fear? Are you in any relationship that brings you sadness or pain?

- Do you hold resentment? Do you have forgiveness?

- How is your self-image? Do you like what you see when you look in the mirror?

- Do you feel healthy and fit? Do you live as a victim of illness?

- Do you have dreams and goals that you are striving for?

- Do you appreciate all that you have around you? Do you take your positive circumstances for granted? Do you give back to those less fortunate? Do you love yourself?

Take time to answer these questions for yourself and look at the answers as a blueprint for your personal healing.

After answering all these questions myself, I tried to put the answers into three boxes or categories. In the first box I put everything about my life, or the past, or my pain situation that I didn't like – things that didn't resonate with me any more, things I wanted to leave behind, for example habits that I needed to break or people I felt were no longer healthy or good for me to be around. I planned to make a few changes in the months ahead, to see if I could tackle some of the issues I wanted to move away from.

In the second box I put the difficulties I was having with my emotions. I wanted to address my feelings as the starting point for my wellness. I needed to dig deeper into the feelings of fear, anger, sadness, shame and so on that I associated with my pain and why it was that I felt I needed to hide my pain or hide my true feelings. So I set myself some themes to work with in my daily journaling. I felt by writing a pain journal I could get the negative emotions, such as anger, out of my head and onto a page.

In the third box I wrote down all the positives I wanted to introduce into my life. I needed to work out a daily wellness plan for myself, concentrating on relaxation, stress management, affirmations, gratitude and the relationship between thoughts and emotions. I decided that my daily journal would be central to this plan. If I was going to commit to writing daily about pain, I needed to balance that with positives, so I would also write a page of things I was grateful for and a list of things I wanted to attract into my life to help my wellness:

- My goal: Self-healing and complete wellness in my body, mind and spirit.

- My intention: I wanted my body to heal itself back to perfect health so I would live in joy and balance.

- My vision: I wanted to live a healthy, full and joyous life, managing my pain or sensations.

So I knew my goal, I set my intention, and then I decided to use a vision board to realise my dream and look at it daily. After all, 'A picture is worth a thousand words.'

Wellness Board

I had heard of vision boards before, and I had read about the law of attraction, i.e. that by focusing on positive thoughts, you bring positive experiences into your life. The theory is that your mind responds strongly to visual stimulation and that by representing your goals with pictures and images, you will actually strengthen and stimulate your emotions, and your emotions are the vibrational energy that activates the law of attraction.

I wanted to draw wellness into my life so I decided to make a wellness vision board to reflect my perfect vision of me. These are so easy to make and can help anchor your goal, remind you of your intention and bring you closer to your vision of a healthier, more positive you in your ideal life. I found it to be a very powerful tool and it really helped me.

What do you need for your wellness vision board?

This is your personal board, you want it to help clarify and maintain your focus on your own health goals. Find pictures that inspire you to create the healthy habits you want to achieve in your new life. So display on your board images of you when you felt happy, or maybe the way you want to feel or look. If you want to return to a hobby, maybe put a picture of that. Or if you have been feeling isolated and want to socialise more or meet someone special, maybe put images of places you would like to go and the kind of people you would like to meet. Your board is very personal: include anything that will help you focus on your wellness – so whatever feels right will be perfect for you.

On my board I had:

- A picture of the last time I did my pain management course when I successfully reduced my medication.

- Lots of beautiful pictures of nature and the outdoors to represent my daily walk.

- A picture of a journal and a pen.

- Pictures of someone meditating.

- Pictures of fruit and water.

Gratitude Board

A gratitude board is exactly what it says on the tin – it shows the things in your life you are grateful for. This sounds simplistic, but research has shown that the simple practice of writing down three things you're grateful for every day for thirty days significantly impacts your sense of appreciation, positivity and satisfaction. I realised from my answers to some of the wellness questions I asked myself as part of my wellness inventory, how easy it was for me to focus on the negatives in my life. Chronic pain can so easily make you look at what is lacking in your life. I often see just the problems, rather than solutions and opportunities. So I decided to practise daily gratitude.

I know I can become agitated easily, retreat into myself, or, worse still, become a constant complainer, as it is so tough constantly battling pain. But I didn't want to let the day-to-day grind of managing pain weigh me down. I wanted to make a conscious effort to actively focus on the good in my life. I wanted to remind myself about all the abundance that surrounds me. I knew I wanted a board that I would see daily, so I used the magnetic board in my kitchen, the heart of the home and the place where I spend most time day to day, and covered it with:

- Pictures of my family, our extended family, friends and my dog.

- Pictures my daughter had painted, special cards from friends and family, anything that I wanted to say 'thank you' for.

I literally counted my blessings and it worked!

News Detox

I wanted to attract only positive energy into my life, so I made another choice. I decided to censor what I watched and listened to on the radio and television. When I was working in the media, I used to read all the daily newspapers, I listened to talk radio and devoured as much news as I could every day. Now, I turned off the news and decided to listen to music I really enjoyed, watch movies that made me laugh and read positive books.

It was a really great experiment; I no longer felt overwhelmed by shocking reports of more doom and gloom. We are constantly bombarded by negative stories; as a nation we seem to thrive on bad news, and it was refreshing not to focus on negativity.

I will say this, though, it isn't as easy as it sounds; you really have to be disciplined not to automatically reach for the phone or computer to see what's going on in the world. So be prepared and organise yourself so that you have feel-good material on your phone that you can listen to or read easily. I had positive podcasts, links to affirmations, healing audio books, songs that made me smile, apps for meditation and even relaxation music all on my phone, and I turned to them each day. It had a hugely positive impact on me during those first few weeks of my wellness plan.

24

Occupational Therapy

Let me preface this chapter by saying that I am in no way an expert on occupational therapy. What follows is an overview of what I did, having worked with an amazing occupational therapist, Blonny Brennan, while on my two pain management courses in St Vincent's Hospital. I knew I had to address how I was living when I embarked on this wellness journey, so, as in the previous chapter, I took an inventory. But before I get to that, let's define what occupational therapy is and why it is so important in the self-management of chronic pain.

The role of the occupational therapist is very important in any hospital treatment plan. They will help you to take control of your life again, manage the long-term effects of pain, and will help you lead a productive, active and fulfilling life. In many respects they provide you with the tools and skills for managing the job of living with pain to enable you to regain your previous lifestyle, as far as that is possible. Your therapist will make an ergonomic assessment of your home or work environment and recommend areas of improvement. You can explore alternatives to your current day-to-day activities and they can work with you to create a healthy, productive and meaningful lifestyle with sustainable results.

As I have mentioned, my personal experience with the wonderful occupational therapist in St Vincent's was very positive and I have learned so much from her. So technically I should know what to do. But pain changes, life changes and we need to adapt to those changes too. So every few months I try to look at my life through the eyes of an occupational therapist.

If you haven't dealt with one on your pain journey so far, I would highly recommend you try to seek out the support of a registered occupational therapist; you might even get a referral from your medical team. They can work with you and the specific needs of your life. Everyone is different and what works for me may not work for you. Often it is tiny changes, little tips and tricks for doing things in an easier way, that make a massive difference.

Taking Control: Pain and the Three Ps

The three Ps to consider are:

- Pacing
- Priorities
- Plan

Pacing

We have mentioned this before, but it is something an occupational therapist can really help you with and it is important to really ask yourself: How could I pace myself in a more productive way?

People tend to save all their energy for the things they really have to do and, because of that, they are often too tired for those activities they enjoy the most. An occupational therapist can show you energy-saving techniques and how to balance your activities throughout the day. It really is about taking the time to manage your pain, to know what activities you can and cannot do, and to learn new ways to do the ones you can't.

Setting up a step-by-step plan will help you to work through the stages and see your progress. The occupational therapist can help you pace certain jobs, maybe by breaking them down into smaller, more manageable tasks. It is important to learn your personal limitations, as these will be different for everyone. Pacing should be applied to all activities, from preparing a meal to decorating a room or doing the weekly shop. It really is about looking at your everyday routine and reassessing it. I have found that a job that I used to do in one day – the weekly shop – is much better for me if I spread it over a number of days. Trying to complete it in one go meant increasing my pain – so I would say to my husband, 'I am just not able!' This negative affirmation, which I was saying often and unconsciously, would soon change too, as I would come to realise the importance of keeping my daily thoughts and beliefs about pain positive.

Priorities

If you can't do everything you want or need to do, how do you know which things you should do?

The answer to this question is a very individual one. You and your occupational therapist will need to talk about it and take into account all the factors involved. For me, my daily walking routine is a priority. Walking helps me reduce stress and tension, which promotes relaxation and, hopefully, sleep.

It is good to chat about a suitable exercise plan with your occupational therapist. Some people feel that if it hurts they are harming themselves more. In fact, if you are less active you weaken your muscles and reduce your endurance, thereby further increasing your pain in the long term.

However, embarking on an exercise plan without medical advice isn't advisable, and everyone's personal situation will be unique, so always get advice. An occupational therapist will suggest ways to gradually build strength and endurance for daily activities and exercise.

Plan

You need to reassess how you live your life and make changes. Part of that can be factoring in time to plan, or taking little steps in preparation for something like a big event. The way you perform leisure and household duties may also aggravate your pain, so you may need to modify things and again this needs planning. An occupational therapist will talk with you about all aspects of your life and look at ways to improve your daily life. But some simple planning really does help.

- **Daily to-do lists:** Break down your day the night before and factor in extra time for each task.

- **Weekly to-do lists:** Prioritise any major tasks that need to be completed and maybe consider doing a little bit every day. Looking at the week ahead can make you really factor in pacing too. Don't take on too much.

- **In-progress to-do lists:** Don't stress about jobs that can be done at any time. You can plan for them, but wait until you are in a good space before tackling things that can be postponed easily.

Plan your Sleep

Sleep is an essential part of our day to ensure we are healthy and ready to engage in what life has to offer. Going to sleep and getting enough sleep are important skills and, often, when you have chronic pain, sleep is the hardest thing to achieve. Sleep is one of the many daily activities that occupational therapy practitioners help to promote. Here are a few tips on getting a better night's sleep that I picked up on my pain management courses:

- Changing your sleeping position with the aid of pillows for support can help to keep pain from disturbing your sleep. You might consider a new mattress, especially if you haven't invested in one in many years.

- Avoid drinking or eating foods that are high in sugar or caffeine in the evening. This proved difficult for me as I like taking my tea and biscuits to bed. Try to drink hot water and lemon instead.

- Wind down, so don't exercise or start to clean the house within one hour of bedtime. I try to read a chapter of a book or read some research on healing and wellness.

- Maintain a good sleep routine. Going to bed and getting up at the same time each day really helps. I know it is really hard when you are struggling with pain, but when I stick to this ritual I find after a week or two the habit is formed and I really feel the benefits – try it.

- While in bed avoid stimulation from television or even the radio, but also, and most important, Facebook and Twitter. Log off social media.

- Listen to the healing relaxation that is free to download with this book (see p. 249) or a guided meditation or relaxing music or some calm nature sounds that help induce sleep. I keep them on my phone and have it beside my bed in case I wake during the night. So instead of getting up and reaching for the remote or checking social media, put your earphones in and R E L A X.

Plan a Return to Work

If chronic pain or recovery from a medical procedure has meant time off work and you are planning your return, I would really recommend that you get some advice from an occupational therapist. A visit to your workplace helps an occupational therapist to understand the difficulties you are experiencing and they will offer advice and make realistic recommendations. For example, a gradual return to work, such as starting part-time and eventually increasing to your regular hours, may be a solution. An occupational therapist can look at your desk and seating position to help you make a successful transition that fits your own personal situation.

Being your own Occupational Therapist Using the Three Ps
Taking Control at Home in Little Steps

I began the process of my occupational therapy inventory around the house. I needed to decide what could work better for me in my life at that moment. So I started with the here and now. It had been over two years since my last pain management course, so I had some adjustments to make.

Here are some of the changes I made in my day-to-day routine. Maybe you can use some of my experience to do your own occupational therapy inventory. You might only make small, simple changes, but I guarantee they can make a big difference.

In the kitchen:

- Rearranging my cupboards at home really helped. I moved all essential items that I used daily into an easily accessible cupboard at eye level, so less bending down or reaching high every day.

- I changed our dishwasher, too. I found that bending down often would trigger spasms in my neck, so I searched for one with a pull-out drawer. Again, no bending down.

- Some other electric appliances were moved to within easy reach for me, so start moving things around to suit your needs and to avoid any unnecessary bending.

- Most importantly, ask for help when you are planning to implement your changes. Talk to your family, and share tasks that you feel add to your pain.

In the living/family room:

- Find a chair that works for you. I often sit on cushions on the floor.

- Over time we have changed our living space to suit my needs. I now have a cosy seating and eating area off the kitchen that is more comfortable for me. My coccyx pain means that I can't sit directly on my bottom so I tend to manoeuvre to the side. Don't underestimate the benefits of a good practical seating.

- A table we often used for breakfast wasn't practical or comfortable for me. We now have a breakfast bar so that I can stand and eat. I became very aware of which sitting positions caused extra stress and pain for me.

- Most recently I have bought a new cordless vacuum cleaner. It is small, light, powerful and I can vacuum while standing, so I don't have to bend, plus it is only charged for 20 minutes so it forces me to stop. Previously I vacuumed on my hands and knees – it was the easiest way to avoid pain, but it was exhausting.

Pain-*free* Life

In the bedroom:

- The big change here was my bed. For years and years I had very low beds, which really didn't help my pain. So now I have a ridiculously high one. I almost need a step up to it, but I don't have to bend to get in.

- Look at different mattress options, invest in some support cushions, anything that will make your sleeping time more enjoyable.

- You could look at other changes, too. For example, I used to keep my shoes in boxes on the floor, so I moved them up to eye level – another way of cutting out bending or reaching for items.

- Making your room a very relaxing, tranquil place will create the right mood for relaxation and sleep. You might consider using an oil burner at night – lavender is always a good choice.

In the bathroom:

- Safety is key for the bathroom! Certain risks can be eliminated and others considerably reduced by simple preventive measures.

- A bath/shower seat can help make you more comfortable and safe while bathing or showering.

- A grab bar is an accessory that can be used in bathtubs and in the shower to reduce the risk of falling and injuring yourself.

- Keep shampoos, conditioners, body wash, etc. on an easy-to-reach shelf, thus avoiding bending.

- Non-slip mats on the inside and outside of the bathtub and shower can help prevent slips and falls.

- Have a safe routine and allow enough time. It's often when you are in a rush that silly accidents happen.

- Take care when washing your hair. This simple act can be a difficult and painful task for many, including myself; so treat yourself at the hairdresser weekly if you can. My other little trick is dry shampoo. Most importantly take care to avoid twists and turns.

The car:

- Test drive: I had a number of very low-to-the-ground, bucket-seat type cars over the years. Of course these were totally impractical for my back. It's the things we do daily, again and again, that can cause increased pain and wear and tear on our bodies. So I decided to test drive a number of cars and I was greatly surprised by the differences in my comfort level.

- Seating position: I had a lot of coccyx pain, so the seating position and height of different cars made a huge difference. For me, a more upright and higher seat was best for back support and put less pressure on my coccyx. And less bending to get into a car has made a massive impact on my pain.

- Automatic: I experienced terrible problems daily pulling up the handbrake and releasing it. I am so grateful that this issue was resolved by switching to an automatic car and already I can feel the benefits.

25

Journaling

'A problem shared is a problem halved.'

Often if we have a problem it can make us feel better just to talk about it to someone who understands. So what happens when there is no one to talk to? Or, as with chronic pain, if it's a problem we don't feel like talking about?

When I embarked on my journey at the start of 2014, I realised I had a lot of anger and bitterness deep inside me because of the burden of pain. To begin my new journey I needed to find a way of dealing with those unresolved feelings. I needed to acknowledge honestly how I felt, so I decided to keep a pain journal. Although later in my journey, as part of my wellness plan, I wanted to refer to my pain as 'sensations', I allowed myself to call it 'pain' in my journal.

I had written diaries since I was a teenager but, in truth, I wasn't always totally honest about my feelings. I needed to pour my raw emotion onto the page: fear, sadness, irritation, anguish, anger, sorrow, shame, grief, aching pain and, in the later journal entries, feelings of trust, joy, confidence and pride in myself. I cannot explain the phenomenon of my pain journal except to say this: it works. And I know it will work for you too.

People are often reluctant to write honestly about what they truly feel, or maybe you might think your spelling and grammar won't be right, but it doesn't matter. I thought I would never show my journal to another human being – it was just for me. Initially, I thought I would just be recording my thoughts, my negative feelings, my mood and my experience with reducing my medication and with my pain management system. I knew what I was going to write wasn't always going to be pretty, and what emerged was far from that. The good, the bad and the ugly all came pouring onto the page.

I had heard many anecdotes about people in therapy writing letters to heal themselves. They would write the letters but not post them, or even burn them. They were using the letters to overcome symbolically whatever it was that they felt was holding them back. And to my surprise and joy I found that it worked! Yes, writing about your pain really is cathartic. *Catharsis* is an ancient Greek word which means purging or cleansing. I took my inspiration from that. This was my way of cleansing my body of the emotions of pain.

That was where the idea came from, the idea of writing down my true feelings about my pain. It was my negative emotion detox. I purged all my gloomy pessimism about my pain onto page after page. I found it highly therapeutic – you can make peace with your darker feelings and the real work of healing can begin.

I started to feel better when I made my pain writing a routine. Often, it seemed, the pages were full of wailing and moaning. But who cares? Once it was out there it was gone and I could focus on my wellness again. But beyond that, with continuous practice, some really amazing breakthroughs happened for me, and I truly experienced a therapeutic cleansing.

At the beginning I would look at the blank page not sure what to write, but I trusted the process of purging my feelings and I wrote. I made an agreement with myself to embrace the act of writing every day and to embrace myself and all my writing in a loving, non-judgemental and compassionate way. All too often I had been very hard on myself, and that harshness needed to be rooted out, for ever. I needed to treat myself as I would a very delicate, sick puppy. Every day I would be gentle and loving – even if the emotions I was writing about were completely the opposite. I accepted that what I wrote came from a place of honesty, that my feelings were valid. But I understood also that those feelings reflected past struggles and didn't belong with the new me. In a very short period of time, I came to a point where I could say: 'I accept those feelings for now but I am not bringing them any further with me on my wellness journey. Their final resting place is here in this journal.'

Writing from a place of self-love and self-care, I experienced remarkable healing and great relief from the words. I was planting the seeds of my healing. The writing was the embarkation point for my healing journey.

So start your journal and you will immediately see the following benefits:

- You are more in contact with your mood and pain level as they fluctuate from day to day, so you can track your progress. It is good to have a daily connection with your pain.

- A routine can be established. Even a little writing is a great achievement in your day. Pain often makes routine difficult.

- It helps to identify when your pain is building, so instead of allowing things to magnify you are tracking small changes in your pain.

- When things rattle around in your mind you can start to 'catastrophise', but by writing things down you can pull back a little and put things into their proper perspective.

- By keeping your journal daily you can read it back at a later date, which is useful for doctor visits.

- Chronic pain can make your memory fuzzy. The daily act of writing things down can translate to other areas of your life and you can become more organised.

- Time spent writing is time for you! You don't have to make any excuses for your feelings, you can just complain if you want to.

- Writing has been proven to alleviate symptoms of stress and depression. It can be a cheap form of self therapy; you can release all your negative thoughts instead of venting at your loved ones.

- By documenting your commitment to wellness you will be more likely to be successful with other positive changes in your life.

- When you are having a bad day you can look back to remind yourself that good days will come again. You can look back over your dreams and hopes for the future and this will make you determined to let the latest flare-up pass and allow you to trust that you will get through the bad day.

There are no hard and fast rules about how to keep a pain journal. All you need to do is choose a notebook. My first one – a bleak school copy book – probably reflected how I was feeling at the time, but it served its purpose. However, I suggest you pick a nice, bright notebook that you love or are drawn to, one you know you will be happy writing in or one that will make you feel uplifted.

In my later journals I got very creative and I would stick things into it, sometimes little uplifting quotes, or pretty pictures, even some recipes and poems! Make sure it is a good size. It doesn't have to be printed with a section or page for each day, but that might help you or encourage you to write every day.

Before I wrote my first entry, I blessed my journal and said aloud that from my writing only good would come. I can be my own harshest critic and I really didn't want this to be a reminder of how badly things were going for me, so I had a few ground rules and you should follow these too:

- Start by adopting a loving, compassionate approach to yourself and accept that everything you write is perfect, no matter what it is.

- Don't ever judge yourself or feel guilty about any emotion you write; your feelings are your true feelings and you must accept them with love.

- Accept as part of your wellness journey that you will have a more balanced life with your body and sensations, so the emotions you write about reflect how you feel now or how you have felt in the past, but don't have to be part of your future.

- On a practical level, write every day, if only for a few minutes. Once you start skipping days, it will be harder and harder to get back to it.

- Write down your reaction to any changes in your daily routine or even any medication changes (always seek medical advice for any change to medications).

- Remember that the way you write is not important. You are writing only for yourself. Don't worry about completing sentences, spelling or word choice. Just get it down on paper or the computer screen!

- Be honest. Write what is true for you. Never judge or censor yourself. This is your journey, so how you are feeling is true for you. If you are struggling with where to start your pain journal, maybe tackle your emotions head on, write about your feelings of anger, fear, anxiety, isolation, guilt etc. and soon you will get into a flow.

- Choose a medium that feels right for you. That could be a special folder on your computer, audio recordings on your phone, a blog or an old-fashioned journal. Do it your way because that's what will work!

- Sometimes it helps to create a comfortable space or a specific time to write your journal. If you can set aside time to do it every day it will probably work better. I always write mine with a lovely cup of tea or a nice biscuit, so choose a favourite corner of your house, in bed, or a place in the sun outside in your garden, whenever feels right for you.

Good luck! I promise you, if you do a little pain journaling every day, in time you will harvest the benefits in your wellness.

26

The Power of Positive Thinking: Affirmations, Autosuggestion and Self-Talk

'The power of positive thinking.' How many times have you heard that phrase? But what does it really mean? What actual 'power' does thinking in a positive way really have? I am sure we'd all agree that thinking positively is a good thing, especially when we're feeling positive and life is going well. However, when you live with chronic pain and are feeling pretty crappy it is a lot harder to stay positive.

I would say I'm a pretty positive person. But I wanted to explore whether actually saying positive affirmations could really change how I was feeling. Could positive thinking change your brain in a physical way? The idea that thoughts can change the structure or function of our brains was discussed by an American, William James, in his 1890 book *Principles of Psychology*. James presented the first theory of neuroplasticity, the term used to describe the brain's ability to change structurally and functionally as a result of personal experience and use.

More recently, neuroscientists have made breakthrough discoveries on how neuroplasticity varies in people with chronic pain. These studies shed new light on how the brain processes pain and could lead to better treatments for chronic pain. The fact that the brain's response to pain can be objectively identified and quantified using brain imaging could lead to improved monitoring and better treatments for chronic pain in the future, and, in turn, to more research.

I started to read more and more about the importance of keeping your thoughts and words positive. The best-selling self-help book, *The Secret* by Rhonda Byrne, is based on the concept of the law of attraction. It explains that you attract into your life whatever you think about. Every thought you think, every word you say, is an affirmation. Even all that private inner dialogue is a stream of affirmations. We are continually affirming and reaffirming subconsciously, with our words and our thoughts, and all these beliefs are creating our life experience in every moment. These beliefs we have are just learned thought patterns, some of which may have been learned in early childhood. And while many of them work well for us, others can work against us. For example, if you are in chronic pain you learn to accept the negative effects of pain, and very often the belief that your pain could flare up leads you to expect catastrophic outcomes.

I wondered what my mind would be capable of if I really applied myself. Could I train my brain to rewire itself or form new neural pathways to stop my pain? I was willing to do the work. Just like exercise, the work required repetition and dedication to reinforce my new mental approach to pain.

First, let's explore affirmation.

Affirmation

An affirmation is usually a short, positive statement in the present tense. It affirms what you desire to be true or something that has already happened. Positive affirmations are used to build a positive internal dialogue. When we consistently repeat positive affirmations, we create positive subconscious thoughts and can make positive changes more quickly and automatically. We are able to create a new positive reality by replacing old and negative thinking with new and positive thoughts. For example:

Every day, in every way, my body is restoring itself to its natural state of perfect health.

When we say an affirmation we think consciously about our words and our thoughts and we must feel them and enjoy them. When we feel positive emotions our mind is instinctively responding to something it believes to be true and we can experience them as true in physical reality. This can be very difficult at first, especially if you are in pain, but I found that repeating my affirmations kept me focused on my inner wellness goals.

An affirmation should reflect your goal and it should include an action component. It should be in the present tense. It should be simple, positive, believable and measurable, and it should carry a reward. A reward is something you desire that works towards your goal, so my reward is feeling good. For example, 'I enjoy how good I feel mentally, physically and emotionally every day.'

At first, it can be strange repeating an affirmation about your health that doesn't seem right, but I found that, over time, continually repeating the affirmation definitely had a positive effect on my overall mood. Affirmations are a way of reprogramming our thought patterns. Change your thoughts – change your life. Could it be that simple?

You should keep your affirmations with you all day, every day, in your purse or wallet, inside your car, typed as a screen saver on your computer, on the fridge or wherever you feel you are most likely to come across them during the day. This enables conscious reinforcement of your affirmations throughout your day. Writing out your affirmations many times can really help the new health goal to make an imprint on your mind. I also found it helped to keep my positive new health affirmation at the forefront of my mind throughout the day. So don't underestimate the power of writing them down. They can be included in your journal so you get into the habit of writing them out daily.

Louise L. Hay, author of the international bestseller *You Can Heal Your Life*, advocates saying and truly feeling your affirmations while looking in the mirror. This can be very effective and powerful as the message is coming from the person we trust most – ourselves! And in the management of chronic pain we are the most important link in the management chain.

When I started out, I chose seven different affirmations, one for each day of the week. I wrote them all down on a huge piece of paper which I stuck on my mirror in my bedroom and practised reading them and trying to really feel them as true. I would repeat them on my morning walk and try constantly to focus on the affirmation.

Say your affirmations with passion, and trust in yourself and your body to heal. When you say them, try to actually feel what it would be like to live pain free; have that feeling of pride, enthusiasm and joy you would feel if you actually lived pain free.

Here's a list of some affirmations that I have picked up from various places and some I have made up for myself. Choose the ones that seem right for you, or make up your own.

- Every cell in my body vibrates with energy and health.

- I am healthy, happy and radiant.

- I believe that all things are possible, and with this under-standing I now create my own vibrant good health.

- As I control my thoughts, I control the way I feel, and I am feeling full of health and vitality.

- My future is safe and secure, I am healthy, I am happy, I am joyful and I am well.

- Gratitude for my body brings love, joy, peace. I naturally attract health and abundance.

- I give thanks for my radiant health and happiness.

- I achieve amazing results with everything I do.

- Loving myself heals my life. I nourish my mind, body and soul.

- I am nourished by the spirit within. Every cell in my body is vibrating with perfect health.

- My body is filled with light. I give thanks for radiant health and endless happiness.

How quickly do affirmations work? It depends on the person. For some people they might even start making a difference from day one. Because affirmations actually re-programme your thought patterns, they change the way you think and feel about things. And because you have replaced dysfunctional beliefs with your own new, positive, healing beliefs, positive change should come easily and naturally – but you need patience.

The important thing to remember is that you must truly believe in the statement. There will be affirmations that resonate with and seem to fit you and you will find you enjoy saying them. These affirmations are likely to be effective for you and hopefully you will start to experience changes almost immediately.

A word of warning, however; affirmations can be positive, but they can also be negative. Try to be aware if you are repeating negative affirmations without thinking. For example, I believed and often unconsciously repeated the affirmations 'I am losing power in my arm' or 'I am just not able'. I said these so often that unknowingly I was making my brain believe they were true.

So watch out for the negative statements you make about your health and try to stop making them.

Autosuggestion
Ask yourself now, 'What limiting beliefs are holding me back?' Answering that question is key to breaking through to the life you really want. A great test is to make a 'Can't' list: a list of what you 'know' you can't do and why.

Complete the following sentence for everything that comes to mind:

I **can't** _____ **because** _____

Pay attention to what comes after the word 'because'. That's your own inner voice telling you that there is a reason this is impossible. That inner voice is what keeps you from being open to any possibility. If a great idea hit you over the head you would instantly dismiss it because you have already decided it's hopeless!

For example, I believed that:

1. 'I **can't** live without pain **because** I have been told by doctors my pain isn't going to go; I will always have it, my pain system is broken.'

2. 'I **can't** live without pain **because** I have a rare condition – Chiari malformation – and constant pain is part of that.'

I had an issue accepting that I would have this pain for ever, so it really resonated with me to think that I could and would heal myself. Replacing the word 'pain' with 'sensations' marked another positive change for me. I decided that from that day on I would believe that I can heal myself; I no longer had pain; I could control my sensations and live free of pain. I needed to challenge my negative beliefs about pain and replace them with positive self-healing beliefs.

Call it brainwashing if you like, but I decided to continually repeat my healing statements with conviction, with trust and a genuine belief in myself and my body to be able to restore balance and wellness. But while I could use these affirmations to alter my conscious mind, how could I make them effective to re-programme my mind on a subconscious level? The answer is by using the technique called autosuggestion. This is the process of training the subconscious mind to believe something it once did not. It is accomplished by repeating affirmations until those statements are internalised. When a person repeats a belief long enough, it sinks into the subconscious and becomes accepted.

When we constantly repeat to ourselves a negative statement, our subconscious mind believes it and it becomes a self-fulfilling prophecy. It becomes manifest in our behaviour. By saying 'I am always in pain', am I programming my mind to experience pain? If autosuggestion is like writing the story of your life, was I writing all about pain? By constantly thinking about pain I was repeatedly telling my subconscious that my life was filled with it. So instead, I had to imagine and create a picture in my mind of what I wanted to have, rather than what I didn't want. Using my wellness board as an aid to visualise my goal was very helpful. I used visualisation to create a movie of my autosuggestion and affirmation goals and I would let my subconscious watch this movie, in which I was an actor playing the part of being pain free.

How can we use autosuggestion to eliminate pain and develop positive good health? We need to programme and condition our mind to make our wellness statement or affirmation into a self-fulfilling prophecy. Autosuggestion should not be practised in a negative way: so instead of saying 'I don't want to have pain', focus on the positive feeling of wellness and what you will do when you are feeling well. When a negative word like 'pain' comes into autosuggestion, it forms a negative picture, which we want to avoid.

Autosuggestion is a repetitive process through which we feed our subconscious with positive statements, positive images and the positive emotions associated with our goal. Repetition alone is not enough. Without visualising the desired outcome, coupled with the positive feelings associated with your goal, it won't work and so will not produce results. Using your wellness board as an aid to visualisation every day can help you to achieve your health goals.

We have all used autosuggestion unconsciously. For example, when you have to catch an early morning flight, you automatically tell yourself that you have got to get up at a certain time. And invariably, you do. A prepared subconscious mind has hunches and gut feelings. After years of telling myself consciously and subconsciously that I was in pain, I knew I would have to focus on a daily routine of controlled positive thoughts, positive visualisation of wellness and focusing every day on what I want more of in life.

Why Saying is Believing: the Science of Self-talk
I realised I needed to engage in positive self-talk. I couldn't believe how much negative self-talk I was using around pain, and it was going on all day on a subconscious level. To my surprise my negative self-talk accounted for as much as 80 per cent of my daily chitter chatter to myself. I challenge you to pay attention

to your self-talk for the next day and see what your self-talk is telling you. What percentage of it is positive, do you think? What percentage of it is negative?

Positive self-talk is the stuff that makes you feel good about yourself and the things that are going on in your life. It is like having an optimistic voice in your head that looks on the bright side, gives you compliments and truly believes in you!

Negative self-talk is the stuff that makes you feel pretty bad about yourself and the things that are going on in your life. This is like having a constant negative voice judging you, telling you that you're not good enough and making you feel pretty miserable.

Being positive all the time isn't achievable – and probably isn't helpful – but maybe self-talk is more than a confidence booster. From a neuroscientific perspective, it might be more like internal remodelling. Self-talk probably does shape the physiology of perception, so could my self-talk help me change the way I perceive pain? I was willing to give it a try.

How can you make your self-talk work for you? We don't always consciously take note of what we're saying to ourselves, but there are a few things you can do to help change the direction of your self-talk:

- Listen to what you're saying to yourself. The first step in improving your self-talk is to actually be aware of what your inner voice is saying. Telling yourself things like, 'I don't think I can do it', 'I can't enjoy my life', 'I can't do that because I will have more pain' are all examples of negative self-talk and can have a negative impact on your psyche.

- Make a conscious effort to think positive. Statements like

'I know I can do it', 'I am filled with positive energy right now' or 'I know I can achieve anything I put my mind to' help your brain pick up the positive cues.

- Monitor your self-talk. Is your self-talk more positive or more negative? Start questioning your self-talk. Ask things like: 'What would I say if a friend were in a similar situation?', 'Is there a more positive way of looking at this?', 'Can I do anything to change what I'm feeling bad about?' Even the simple act of monitoring your self-talk can be a useful exercise to see how you deal with different situations.

- Change your self-talk. Consciously change the negative self-talk into positive self-talk. It's easier said than done, but definitely worth working on. When you notice negative self-talk, say to yourself, 'No. Stop', and replace the negative thought with a positive statement. For example, if you think, 'I'll never be able to do this', ask yourself 'Is there anything I can do that will help me be able to do this?' Believe in yourself and trust that everything is working out for your good.

- You can use self-talk to motivate yourself. Motivational self-talk means using encouraging phrases like, 'Come on!', 'Let's go!', 'You can do this', 'You will do your walk today.' You can also use it to help you achieve what you want. Instructional self-talk is helpful when practising a task like journaling. You instruct yourself until it becomes automatic. For example, you might tell yourself, 'Write one page before noon', or 'You will see the benefits from saying your wellness affirmations daily'.

Keep your self-talk short, precise and consistent. If the thought isn't as positive as you would like, reverse the thought and consciously start forming new neural pathways for new, positive thoughts. If you find it hard to say positive things to yourself, maybe write down some examples and get into the habit of saying them. The more you work on improving your self-talk the better you will get. Like starting anything new, it won't be easy at first, but it will get better with time.

No matter what you call your inner statements, you're instructing your subconscious mind on what you want. You do this either consciously or subconsciously, deliberately or habitually. The only way to change those directives, and their results, is to change what you say to yourself through affirmations, autosuggestion and self-talk. Consistently focus your mind on what you want, with positive statements, affirmations and images of your wellness and good health – you are destined to achieve them.

Who knew talking to yourself could change your life? Believe me, this *will* change your life.

27

The Power of Your Mind to Heal

I had heard about the placebo effect, but I didn't really understand the importance of it or why it could be relevant to me and my wellness. I knew it involved giving someone a fake procedure or sugar pill that they believed to be a real medical treatment; the patient's condition would improve because they had an expectation that it would. This magical 'healing' is well documented in many clinical trials. However, I had also heard sad stories of people dying because they were given the placebo drug, so I didn't have much faith in its application until I began to research it.

One of the most illuminating pieces of research into the placebo effect that I found was a fascinating TEDx talk on healing by an American doctor called Lissa Rankin, who spoke about the power of our thoughts. Did you know that if you think negative thoughts, your brain releases chemicals associated with those thoughts? There is an extreme difference between the chemicals that are released with a positive thought and those released with a negative thought. Positive thoughts create joy, good health, and so on. Negative thoughts create undesirable situations and events in our lives, and can even create disease. This is the dark shadow side of the placebo – it's called the 'nocebo' effect. If a patient is told that they might experience negative symptoms in response to the treatment or sugar pill, this becomes a self-fulfilling prophecy. Some patients who believed they were receiving chemotherapy actually lost their hair!

Could it be that simple? Can your mind heal your body with thoughts alone? And if so, what medical and scientific evidence exists to prove it? Exploring this led me to the Institute of Noetic Sciences (IONS). Founded in 1973 by Apollo 14 astronaut Edgar Mitchell, it is, to quote its website (www.noetic.org), a 'non-profit research, education and membership organization whose mission is supporting individual and collective transformation through consciousness research, educational outreach, and en-gaging a global learning community in the realization of our human potential'. IONS researches the potential and power of consciousness, exploring phenomena that do not necessarily fit conventional scientific models.

IONS document a fascinating piece of research called the Spontaneous Remission Project. In this work, the authors, Caryle Hirshberg and the late Brendan O'Regan, defined spontaneous remission as 'the disappearance, complete or incomplete, of a disease or cancer without medical treatment or treatment that is considered inadequate to produce the resulting disappearance of disease symptoms or tumour'. The Spontaneous Remission Project catalogued the world's medical literature on the subject and the resulting book was the largest database in the world of medically reported cases of spontaneous remission, with more than 3,500 references from more than 800 journals in twenty different languages.

What is spontaneous remission? Could it be instantaneous healing? In medical terms, the term 'spontaneous', as it relates to remission, is used for a significant and measurable reduction in tumour size, or a reversal in the progression of a disease, and when this improvement cannot be attributed to Western allopathic medical treatment. While researching the concept of spontaneous healing I came across a case study that really resonated with me.

The patient at the centre of the study, a young American girl, suffered from crippling rheumatoid arthritis, yet it appeared that she had somehow healed her illness with hypnotherapy. I felt I could identify with some of the symptoms associated with this illness and I couldn't help but wonder, 'Do I have the power to heal myself?'

I began to explore all types of spontaneous healing. I was intrigued when I read about scientifically proven real-life medical 'miracles' relating to the sudden and complete cure of a disease without medical treatment. The phenomenon at Lourdes is a good example of this. Is it the hand of God or the power of faith that has cured so many people at the famous Marian shrine there? Since the apparitions in 1858, Lourdes has reported about seven thousand cases of unexplained cures. In 1883 a body called the *Bureau des Constatations Médicales* began documenting all cases. This was the forerunner to the International Medical Committee of Lourdes (CMIL), founded in 1947, which is made up of around twenty members, each respected in their own particular area of medical expertise. This committee makes judgements about cases reported to them. One or more of its members examine each case in detail. They read up on all the medical literature published on related subjects and may consult with colleagues outside the CMIL. Once a year the committee votes on whether to accept or refuse to confirm that the various cures reported to them are inexplicable according to present scientific knowledge. A two-thirds majority is required for an affirmative vote. This rigorous process has deemed that (as of July 2013) sixty-nine cases were considered to be miracles.

Can the Brain Affect the Body at a Cellular Level?

It seems that your attitude really does matter. If you have a positive mindset, your positive brain can affect your body. Expectations are powerful, so could my positive thoughts alone be enough to heal my pain system? Can I create my own placebo effect?

Positive thoughts in your brain communicate through hormones and neurotransmitters. Negative thoughts are interpreted by the part of the brain called the amygdala as a threat, which makes the adrenal glands trigger the 'fight or flight' stress response. (The 'fight or flight' response was first described by Harvard physiologist Walter Bradford Cannon.) Fight or flight, which is hardwired into our brains, is a genetic wisdom designed to protect us from bodily harm. The response actually originates from an area of the brain called the hypothalamus. When the hypothalamus is stimulated it initiates a sequence of nerve cell firing and chemical release that prepares our body for running or fighting.

The good news is that I discovered that our bodies also have a relaxation response, which we can learn to switch on and harvest the benefits for our own healing and well-being. The term 'relaxation response' was coined by Herbert Benson, who founded Harvard's Mind/Body Medical Institute. This response is defined as your personal ability to encourage your body to release chemicals and brain signals that make your muscles and organs slow down and increase blood flow to the brain. In his book *The Relaxation Response* Benson describes the scientific benefits of relaxation. The parasympathetic nervous system switches on, sending out healing hormones to our body. Extensive research has shown that regular practice of the relaxation response can be an effective treatment for a wide range of stress-related disorders and health problems.

The many methods of eliciting the relaxation response include visualisation, progressive muscle relaxation, energy healing, acupuncture, massage, breathing techniques, prayer, meditation,

Reiki, tai chi, qigong and yoga. According to Herbert Benson, one of the most valuable things we can do in life is to learn deep relaxation – making an effort to spend some time every day quieting our minds in order to create inner peace and better health. Give yourself the permission to explore ways to truly relax every day, treat your precious body with loving care, listen, connect and believe in your own self-repair mechanisms to heal.

Taking all my research on board I was faced with the question of how I was going to harness the relaxation response in my daily life to boost my own internal healing and pain management. My search would bring me back to my brain and the power of my own subconscious mind. I have to admit my decision to formally study hypnotherapy came from a deep internal knowledge that it would work. I had already experienced some triumphs with my homemade version of hypnosis, and I had an inner belief that seemed to guide me into the unknown depths and power of my unconscious mind. I felt my body was whispering to me to just do it!

28

My Healing Relaxation Hypnosis

In this final chapter I want to share with you something I devised specifically to help me with pain. It is the 'healing relaxation hypnosis' that accompanies this book and is free for you to use as part of your daily wellness programme.

I want to start by saying that hypnotherapy isn't a miracle cure for pain relief and I don't make any such claims. But I do want to provide you with some background to how my slightly unorthodox method came about and show you how I got this to work for me and how I hope you can make it work for you. I will also tell you about a method for self-hypnosis based on the principles of Émile Coué (1859–1926), a French psychologist and pharmacist, author of *Self Mastery through Conscious Autosuggestion*, and known as the 'prophet of autosuggestion'.

After I finished my sessions with the Goldin Clinic and I began using my own homemade relaxation hypnosis recordings (which I describe in chapters 19 and 21), my continuing research kept bringing me back to the whole area of hypnosis. I discovered that there is scientific proof that hypnotism really does have a measurable impact on the brain. A study by one of America's leading psychiatrists, David Spiegel of Stanford University, scanned the brains of hypnotised volunteers who were told they were looking at coloured objects when, in fact, the objects were black and white. A scan showing areas of the brain used to register colour highlighted increased blood flow, indicating that the volunteers genuinely 'saw' colours, as they had been told they would. 'This is scientific evidence that something happens in the brain when people are hypnotised that doesn't happen ordinarily,' said David Spiegel. It is a fascinating study and definitely worth reading.

After much consideration and because I truly believe in the power of the mind in pain management, I decided to train with Niamh Flynn and study the science of hypnosis. I really enjoyed my training; it was so much fun being a student again, and I met some amazing people on the course, who have become friends. We shared ideas and our innermost thoughts and we all success-fully passed our exams in November 2014. I was now a certified clinical hypnotherapist with the National Guild of Hypnotists.

My appetite for knowledge and learning continued to grow and by the end of the year I was in London studying angel card reading with Doreen Virtue and Radleigh Valentine. I had used angel cards daily for many years and choosing a card was part of my daily wellness routine, so I thought, 'Why not study something I really enjoy?' I was having fun and exploring things I wouldn't have thought possible at the start of the year. What a difference a year had made in my life. As another new year dawned I continued with my tradition of writing down my goals and burying them in the soil so that they would grow and bloom and, once more, I burned anything that no longer served me.

At the start of 2015 I felt I still had more to learn and explore. I tried to use the principles of hypnosis and combine them with other alternative healing methods. It was my determination to find a way of reducing my pain 'sensations' naturally that kept me searching for the right method for me. I was constantly trying to devise different scripts, using different guided visualisations, of longer or shorter duration, to get the perfect healing relaxation hypnosis for my own personal use. I made so many over a period of months. It's fortunate that I work in the sound business – I made great use of the home studio. When I got a formula I was happy with, some good friends (with and without pain) and family members kindly listened to them and would report back if they felt they were useful to them.

Things changed for me again when I decided to explore Reiki as part of my journey to wellness. Reiki is a Japanese technique for stress reduction and relaxation that also promotes healing. The name comes from two Japanese words: *Rei*, which means 'God's wisdom' or the 'higher power', and *Ki*, which means 'life-force energy'. So Reiki is actually 'spiritually guided life-force energy'. It is generally administered by 'laying on hands' and is based on the idea that an unseen 'life-force energy' flows through us and is what causes us to be alive.

I began training with a wonderful teacher called Aidan Storey, the bestselling author of *On Angels' Wings* and *Angels of Divine Light*, and a gifted healer and Reiki master. I instantly connected with the principles of Reiki. After beginning my study of Reiki, my hypnosis healing went up to a different level and I felt I had the perfect relaxation tool. True to form, I recorded many versions. I felt that by harnessing the power of the subconscious mind with the principles of hypnosis, merging it with the essence of Reiki healing, and drawing on the healing angels, I had the perfect combination for me. I still use this method daily to manage my pain sensations and bring balance and positivity into my day. I have devised various different versions that I use for all areas of my life.

I think you will find my healing relaxation hypnosis a great tool to help you on your wellness journey. To start, try to commit to using it day and night for twenty-one days. Most people believe that completing a task for twenty-one days in a row forms habits. In addition to using my hypnosis, I would also encourage you to follow the easy steps to learn 'self-hypnosis'.

Hypnosis: a Practical Method of Pain Management

I have had great success personally with hypnosis, and I truly believe that a good hypnotherapist can help you make permanent and positive changes in your life. If you see one regularly they can help you get into hypnosis deeper and faster than you may be able to on your own. However, sessions with a hypnotherapist are not cheap, so I want to share the concept of self-hypnosis.

Self-hypnosis has not only helped me reduce my pain and sleep better, it has also eased my daily stress about living in pain. I first tried self-hypnosis while I was studying, so I had lots of time to get advice from my brilliant teacher Niamh and I managed to perfect my technique to get optimum results. I now use it twice a day, morning and evening, and occasionally I use it during the day as well or if I wake during the night.

I believe that self-hypnosis can work for you as part of your pain management programme. It is cost-effective and easy to learn, but you will have to spend some time learning to perfect it. I believe it is worth the small investment in time because each time you practise self-hypnosis, you'll go further down, and the deeper you go, the better it works. I truly believe that we all have the ability, with practice, to hypnotise ourselves and tap into the power of our own subconscious mind. Initially I didn't really have any concept of how powerful our subconscious is. In pain management, I have discovered, it is a great ally in achieving a reduction in our pain sensations. All you need to do is learn how to utilise it and you will achieve a great deal.

Pain-*free* Life

A quick overview

- Hypnosis is a relaxed state of attentive concentration that allows your conscious, critical mind to rest temporarily, so that you can be receptive to positive thoughts that help you to feel more comfortable. In this relaxed state of attentive concentration, you are helped to use your own imagination to change your experience in a way that is acceptable, desirable and pleasant for you.

- Hypnosis is not a sleeping state. When you are in hypnosis, you are awake and alert, but you feel deeply and pleasantly relaxed. And when you are deeply relaxed, you cannot feel uncomfortable. It is a trance state, characterised by extreme suggestibility, relaxation and heightened imagination. So contrary to what you might think, it is not really like sleep, because you are in control and alert the whole time. It is most often compared to daydreaming, or the feeling of 'losing yourself' in a book or movie. You are fully conscious, but you tune out most of the stimuli around you. You focus intently on the subject at hand, virtually to the exclusion of any other thought.

- Hypnosis is great for pain control because when you are deeply relaxed in hypnosis, you cannot be uncomfortable. That is because relaxation is the opposite of discomfort. When you are deeply relaxed, you can filter out uncomfortable sensations and tune into the experience of other, more comfortable, sensations.

- In hypnosis, the door to your subconscious mind opens, so that, with your permission, your subconscious mind can retrieve the information it needs to help you to become more comfortable. And you can learn to do this on your own. This is what makes hypnosis such an excellent tool for pain management and for relieving discomfort.

- Hypnosis works best for appropriately medically diagnosed physical pain. In other words, we should *not* use hypnosis to get rid of acute pain that signals that there is a medical condition that needs to be fixed. We do not want to mask a correctable medical problem.

- We do want to use hypnosis to get rid of all unnecessary pain and discomfort that has been medically determined to be unnecessary. Hypnosis is also effective with discomfort that has strong psychological or emotional aspects.

Self-hypnosis

The first rule of self-hypnosis is – remember to be positive! In hypnosis it is very important to be careful about what we focus on. Our subconscious mind favours what we really want. So it's good to focus on what we want to attract into our day-to-day life, instead of what we don't want. For example, if you don't want to get ill or have more pain, focus on perfect health. The idea is to be positive because the mind is designed to be optimistic, and negative or fearful thoughts will only attract more of the same into our lives. So start with a positive mindset.

The Coué Method

'One must not be a slave, but the master of one's subconscious mind.'

Émile Coué is famous for his mantra-like conscious auto-suggestion, 'Every day, in every way, I am getting better and better.' If you are overwhelmed with pain sensations, it can be very difficult to think and speak positively all the time. When you start to practise autosuggestion every day you can, as far as possible, start to rework the negative thoughts as they arrive.

However, with hypnosis you are working with your sub-conscious mind. The subconscious mind is the record keeper of everything you have experienced in your life, it drives your behaviour without thought – thinking is the job of your conscious mind. During self-hypnosis your mind must truly believe the wellness affirmations that you are repeating, so tailor make them to be true for you. The subconscious mind is the key player for success, as we are trying to reprogramme it to download this new belief. It is important to say your affirmations to yourself, not only at the conscious level but, even more importantly, at the subconscious level – and really the only way to reach the subconscious is with hypnosis and deep relaxation.

I believe my daily application of both conscious and sub-conscious autosuggestions or affirmations is the secret to my healing. My first 'Aha!' moment of realisation, inspiration and insight about the value of self-hypnosis was when I understood that the subconscious mind is always listening to our self-talk. The subconscious cannot tell the difference between what is real or imagined. It makes perfect sense when you think of our reactions to a scary movie – it makes us scared, it feels real. At a conscious level the mind knows it's just a movie, but the subconscious doesn't so we feel fear.

I followed the Coué method for three weeks, three times a day – on waking, once during the day and just before I went to sleep – I also wrote down my affirmation ten times a day, and said it regularly throughout the day. I really applied myself to it for a week and something shifted mentally. If you commit to this practice for twenty-one days, I believe you will see results.

Here's what to do:

The Technique: Week 1

1. In bed, just before you are ready to fall asleep and (if you want) again when you first wake but are still feeling sleepy, repeat the following suggestion ten times: 'Every day, in every way, I am getting better and better.' (You could choose another suggestion. I used: 'I release all chronic pain from my body now, I merely have sensations and I can control all the sensations in my body'. Alternatively, make up your own.)

2. While you are saying the suggestion, think, feel and imagine yourself getting better and better, try to actually feel better, have the feeling in your core with every repetition. Remain serious about your goal and believe it will happen.

3. In order not to fall asleep and not to lose count every time you say the suggestion press down with each finger on your right hand. Then, continue with each finger of your left hand until you've completed the suggestion ten times.

If you start to daydream during this process, start again and keep going until you've finished ten consecutive counts. This may be your first attempt at learning to programme yourself through suggestion, but persist.

It is of the utmost importance to do this exercise every night without falling asleep and without interruption until you've completed the ten repetitions. I increased it to twenty-five repetitions in the first week and you might want to try that too. Although for the first week you only have to do the evening exercise, if you can, follow the same pattern in the morning and during the day. This is the foundation for establishing a habitual pattern of programming yourself by giving yourself positive suggestions and affirmations. It is really powerful if you do this before falling asleep and when you wake because at these times your mind is already in a trance-like state.

This really works. You'll find yourself reacting very positively to your suggestion and if you use your own affirmations and suggestions over the coming weeks, it is a habit that will make an enormously positive change to your life.

The Technique: Week 2 – basic induction

1. Continue the pre-sleep (and waking) technique you learned in the first week. If you have only been practising it once a day it is important that you now start to do it both morning and night. So twice a day say your affirmation, 'Every day, in every way, I am getting better and better.'

2. In addition, this week do the following: twice a day, once in the morning or at noon, and once in the early evening, hypnotise yourself, stay in hypnosis for two to three minutes, and then wake yourself up. If you think you can't do it, trust me: it is very simple if you follow the following technique. Just think of it as a mini-meditation or focused relaxation.

    *   Sit in a comfortable chair with your back supported, or lie on your bed or couch if that is more comfortable. Focus your attention effortlessly on a spot opposite you, slightly above eye level.

    *   Slowly take three deep breaths. Each time, when you inhale, hold it for the mental count of four full seconds as you count backwards: four ... three ... two ... one.

    *   Close your eyes, exhale, *relax*, and allow yourself to go into a deep hypnotic rest.

3. Remain in a hypnotic state for approximately two to three minutes by counting down slowly from twenty-five to one. Visualise each number being written on a blackboard and as you count backwards imagine rubbing the number away. Have a mental picture of the numbers and see yourself carefully rubbing off the number as you count backwards. Between each count and before you imagine seeing the next number, say your affirmation for that week: 'Every day, in every way, I am getting better and better.' Then simply imagine drawing the next number, imagine rubbing it off and say your affirmation again. I found that my mind wandered a lot at the beginning and when it did, I started again (if I had the time), and this might work for you too.

4. To awaken, when you have reached the number one, take three deep breaths, hold the last one for the mental count of four and then just count forwards from one to four. I would say to myself that I was going to awaken refreshed and alert, ready to go about my business in an energetic way.

5. Do this exercise twice a day for seven days, after which you will be ready to give yourself beneficial suggestions.

The Technique: Week 3 – programmed suggestion
After successfully following the instructions for weeks one and two, you are ready to start the third step of self-hypnosis. You will need some paper and a pen and some card or paper. I would recommend that you buy some cards as you will need to carry them around with you all the time. Use whatever will work for you and is durable enough to last for the week.

On your card, write a simple goal that is specific, measurable, action-oriented, achievable, realistic, time-bound and written in the present tense, so that your mind will believe that it *is* true for you. A good example would be: 'I am working on my wellness every day. I do this by walking twenty minutes every day and listening to my relaxation hypnosis in the morning and night, and I write about my wellness journey in my journal every evening.' The more specific the goal the easier it is for your mind to move in the direction it needs to achieve it.

You can continue to do step one, saying your affirmation ten times: 'Every day, in every way, I am getting better and better.' This is a perfect way to relax your mind and body before starting step three. For the next step you need clear your mind of any thoughts and allow yourself five minutes alone for peaceful relaxation.

As in step two, sit down and choose a spot opposite you, slightly above eye level. Begin with your breathing. Slowly take a deep breath and, as you inhale, hold it for four full seconds as you count backwards: four ... three ... two ... one. Allow your mind to *relax*.

Repeat this until your mind is calm and ready to focus. Then hold the card in front of the spot and read the suggestion to yourself three times: 'I am working on my wellness every day. I do this by walking twenty minutes every day and listening to my relaxation hypnosis in the morning and night, and I write about my wellness journey in my journal every evening.' (If you want, you can also include your affirmation: 'Every day, in every way, I am getting better and better.' If you don't feel the card will work for you, get a large piece of paper and write out the goal and stick the paper on a spot opposite to you. I did this in my bedroom so I could read my goal every time I passed it during the day).

Make sure the words on the card are believable to you. Allow yourself to imagine accomplishing what is written on the card. Use your imagination to visualise everything on the card in great detail. After reading the suggestion to yourself three times, either drop the card or focus on it as you take another deep breath. Exhale. Take your second deep breath. Exhale.

Now, take your third deep breath and hold it for the mental count of four. Close your eyes as you count backwards: four … three … two … one. Exhale, and go into deep hypnosis.

Repeat the mantra and as you do so, imagine a big movie screen. On the screen see yourself carrying out each suggestion. See yourself getting ready for your walk, maybe see the road or park where you will walk every day, what you are wearing, the time of day you will take your walk. Then imagine where you will listen to your relaxation tape etc., visualise it in great detail on the imaginary cinema screen and continue to repeat the mantra.

You'll find that at times the words start to break up and become fragmented. That's perfectly okay. The important words or phrases will come through to you.

If you find the cinema screen too difficult and you are more comfortable with the established method in step two, use the numbers on the blackboard method, counting backwards from twenty-five to one. As the numbers disappear, allow the suggestion to repeat over and over in your subconscious mind. Between rubbing out one number and going on to the next, imagine for a moment that you are carrying out your suggestion.

In two or three minutes you'll have a feeling that it's time to stop and wake up. This time was set when you established a habit pattern in step two. So don't worry too much about it – you can stop whenever feels right for you.

At this point, clear your imaginary screen, take a deep breath, and count forward: one … two … three … four. Now open your eyes and go about your day. I try to say something positive at this point. If you want to try this, you can say it aloud or internally: 'I am feeling refreshed and relaxed in every way. Today is going to be a good day.'

Give yourself time to allow the suggestions to take hold. It can take up to two weeks to start experiencing the benefits related to your suggestions.

Self-hypnosis: Quick Tips

- Self-hypnosis can be used for so many areas of your life – self-confidence, self-esteem, goal setting, weight loss, in work, anything you want to achieve.

- Before you begin, decide how you will present your suggestions or health goal to yourself. You may want to write out your suggestions before you begin.

- If you are using self-hypnosis to manage pain with the aim of reducing the amount of medication you're on, talk to your GP. You may have great success if you practise self-hypnosis daily, but before you decide to reduce or stop taking medication *always* talk to your healthcare practitioner and get advice. *Never* alter your medication schedule without the explicit instructions of your healthcare practitioner.

- There's no right or wrong time to perform self-hypnosis. One of the most effective times, though, is shortly before you go to sleep at night. The process of deliberately inducing relaxation helps you to fall asleep faster and get a better night's sleep. You'll also find that the affirmations, repeated shortly before bedtime, will be absorbed by your subconscious mind quickly and easily.

Every time you practise self-hypnosis, you'll find you can go deeper. It will be easier and faster to get into self-hypnosis each time you do it, so practise your self-hypnosis skills every day. You can use my free hypnosis that accompanies this book to help you deal with daily pain and to keep you focused on wellness. To access the free hypnosis just go to www.andreahayes.ie/media and use the password 'healing hypnosis'.

Final Thoughts

The most important thing in any journey to wellness is to trust your instincts and do what is best for you medically, physically, emotionally and spiritually. Work with your medical team but, remember, you are the most important person in the team. You have the key to unlock the door to your pain-free life. Ignore the opinions of others – they have no idea what you have to go through – and do what is best for you.

If you have difficulty sleeping, try sleeping at different times of the day or night. Sleep is restorative and important for your health. If you are not sleeping, at least rest and put on the relaxing hypnosis that accompanies this book or find a good meditation CD to help with mind and body healing.

Remember that you are not alone. Please reach out to me and others like me who know what you are dealing with. Allow family and friends to help. You can't do it all alone – we all need support, and by sharing the burden everyone benefits.

Work towards developing a positive new attitude to your life and the management of your pain. Create the plan that works for you. You are important, so live your life to the fullest and with abundance.

Here are some daily reminders and planning that should help you on your journey:

- Plan time to listen to the healing hypnosis that you can download (see p. 249) or any relaxing recording or meditation.

- Plan time for affirmations and autosuggestion.

- Plan journaling – write your pain and gratitude pages.

- Find the right support.

- Stay positive. Chronic pain can always be managed.

- Remember, you have the right to effective treatment. Seek out a medical team that gives you the care you need.

- Remember pacing and spacing daily, and allow yourself to rest in between activities.

- Be confident that you will find the relief from chronic pain that you seek.

- Remember that you are not alone. Share your pain. Seek help from chronic pain support groups.

Chronic pain affects more than 1.5 billion people worldwide. Fortunately, advances in research have found some of the ways in which chronic pain changes the brain, and several promising research areas could lead to better treatment approaches.

I have decided to be my own 'cure'. I have taken the power back and have become an empowered patient. I wish you blessings of health and wellness on your journey. Consider what a long way you've come *today*! We may be judged, we may not be believed, but believe this – you have your own innate ability to heal yourself, so trust yourself.

When I am feeling down and maybe even a little crazy I remember, 'The tallest oak in the forest was once just a little nut that held its ground.' They may call us nuts, but hold your ground and don't give up!

Epilogue

In July 2015, after many months of feeling very unsteady and faint when standing up, I went for a diagnostic tilt table test in the Mater Hospital in Dublin and it was confirmed I have a condition called postural orthostatic tachycardia syndrome or POTS. I am managing that now through adjustments to my diet and lifestyle and I am on reduced medication to try to alleviate some side effects of this condition, which has already helped. With any medication changes comes adjustment and patience – I am not completely medication free but am aiming to be in the future.

I continue to receive intermittent pain procedures with Dr. Murphy in St Vincent's Hospital and my recent scans have been reviewed once again by Dr Ashley Poynton in the Mater Hospital. He has suggested a surgical option to treat the degenerative disc disease and foraminal stenosis in my cervical spine. We have discussed an anterior cervical discectomy, decompression and fusion to remove the discs between vertebrae C5/C6 and C6/C7, thereby decompressing the nerve roots. The neck would be reconstructed using underbody cages and a plate with six screws. The purpose of this surgery is to address my neck and bilateral arm pain. As with any surgery the outcome cannot be predicted, and it may not address my upper cervical pain and headaches – Dr Poynton feels these are most likely due to the Chiari malformation, the surgical option for which is decompression brain surgery. At the time of finishing this book I am still strongly considering each option and continue to work on my own pain management strategies to minimise the pain.

In September 2015 I was appointed to the governing body of

the Irish charity Chronic Pain Ireland and I am honoured to have been part of their first multi-disciplinary pain management pilot programme in Ireland, where I outlined my pain management programme related in this book and received wonderful feedback from the patients.

I continue to work on advocacy for the awareness of chronic pain conditions and invisible illness. It is my hope that this book will play a part in getting the message out to a wider audience and that soon none of us suffering from chronic pain will have to do so in silence for fear of ridicule and disbelief.

Further Reading

Brand-Miller, Jennie, *The New Glucose Revolution Guide To Living Well With PCOS* (Hachette Livre, Australia, 2004)

Byrne, Rhonda, *The Secret* (Atria Books, New York, 2006)

Coué, Émile, *Self Mastery Through Conscious Autosuggestion* (Allen & Unwin, London, 1923)

Harris, Colette and Theresa Cheung, *PCOS Diet Book: How You Can Use The Nutritional Approach To Deal With Polycystic Ovary Syndrome* (Thorsons, London, 2002)

Hay, Louise L., *You Can Heal Your Life* (Hay House, Carlsbad, 1984)

James, William, *The Principles of Psychology* (Henry Holt and Co., New York, 1890)

Rankin, Lissa, *Mind Over Medicine: Scientific Proof That You Can Heal Yourself* (Hay House, Carlsbad, 2013)

Speigel, David and Spiegel, Herbert, *Trance And Treatment: Clinical Uses Of Hypnosis* (2nd revd edition, American Psychiatric Press Inc., Arlington, 2004)

Storey, Aidan, *Angels Of Divine Light* (Transworld, Dublin, 2010)

Storey, Aidan, *On Angels' Wings* (New Island, Dublin, 2011)

Trickett, Shirley, *Coping With Candida: Are Yeast Infections Draining Your Energy?* (Sheldon Press, London, 1994)

Vernon, Michael and Shepperson Mills, Dian, *Endometriosis: A Key To Healing And Fertility Through Nutrition* (Thorsons, London, 2002)

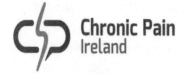
Chronic Pain
Ireland

If you are not your own doctor, you are a fool.
Hippocrates (*c.* 460–400 BC)

Chronic Pain Ireland provides support and information to those living with chronic pain while working with all the major stakeholders. CPI provides a range of services, including self-management workshops which are held nationwide. In addition the organisation produces a quality newsletter and provides telephone and website support.

The workshops on self-management techniques are the most important aspect of the work we do. The workshops are critically important for those who have been through a pain management programme or attended a pain management clinic. People living with chronic pain at a moderate to severe level require access to a multi-disciplinary team and in particular support from family and friends.

The objectives of our self-management courses are to improve the quality of life of the person living with chronic pain, reduced pain sensation, reduced and more appropriate use of medications and in some cases a return to employment. Recent research indicates that a 'mind–body' approach to self-management is essential if it is to succeed. In other words you cannot separate the psychological treatment from the physiological treatment of the patient.

CPI has now embarked on a new programme of self-management taking on board the latest thinking in dealing with chronic pain using the mind-body approach. These programmes will be audited to assess their effectiveness and it is hoped that the new programme will be rolled out nationwide.

Andrea Hayes is living proof that the 'mind–body' approach works. Her book will be an inspiration to all who have struggled over many years to cope with their chronic pain and should be read by all living with chronic pain and in particular by healthcare professionals.

John Lindsay
Chairperson, Chronic Pain Ireland